The Ultimate Guide
to Strap-on Sex

Ultimate Guides from Cleis Press

The Ultimate Guide to Anal Sex for Women
by Tristan Taormino

The Ultimate Guide to Pregnancy for Lesbians
by Rachel Pepper

The Ultimate Guide to Strap-on Sex
by Karlyn Lotney

The Ultimate Guide to Strap-on Sex

A Complete Resource for Women and Men

KARLYN LOTNEY

CLEIS
PRESS

Published in the United States by Cleis Press Inc., P.O. Box 14684, San Francisco, California 94114.

Printed in the United States.
Cover design: Scott Idleman
Text design: Karen Quigg
Logo art: Juana Alicia
First Edition.
10 9

The publisher wishes to thank Tristan Taormino, whose *The Ultimate Guide to Anal Sex for Women* launched the Ultimate Guide series from Cleis Press.

Illustrations on pages 9, 18, and 91 by MB Condon are reprinted from *The New Good Vibrations Guide to Sex: Tips and Techniques from America's Favorite Sex Toy Store* by Cathy Winks and Anne Semans (Cleis Press, 1997). Copyright 1997 by Cathy Winks and Anne Semans. Illustrations on pages 39, 40, 42, and 87 are reprinted with permission of Stormy Leather. Illustration on page 101 is reprinted with permission of Vixen Creations.

This book is dedicated to Kyra Michelle Miller,

the ultimate guide to my heart.

Acknowledgments

I would like to extend my heartfelt thanks to a bunch of people who have encouraged me and have contributed to the creation of this book. My parents, Barbara and Kenneth Lotney, have gone over and above the call of duty in lending their early morning encouragement, unfailing understanding, and unconditional love. To LaTricia Ransom and Shannon Lee Turner who devoted time, energy and tremendous talent to reading and commenting on the manuscript. To all of my friends, especially Liz Miller-Pastore, Molly McKay, Hima B., Rebecca Goldfader, and spouses, Angie, Davina and A, for their loving encouragement and solidarity through my hermit phases, and to Leslie Einhorn, for her inestimable support and nearly nightly peer counseling sessions. To Don Weise, Felice Newman, Frédérique Delacoste of Cleis Press for publishing this manuscript and to copyeditor Liz Highleyman. To all of my amazing interns, Liz, Kathryn, Gloria, Kristin, Rez, Sara and Lyndsey, for their general assistance and for their generous, committed efforts toward this book, and to my inspiring workshop participants as they continue to refine my understanding of sexuality. To some of my heroes and fellow sex educators, Staci Haines, Carol Queen, Annie Sprinkle, Jackie and Shar, Joani Blank, Skeeter, Susie Bright, Jack Morin, and all of my Good Vibrations coworkers. To good friends Robert, Brenda, Alicia, Janine, Alison, Stephanie R., Nini, Laurel Sharp and Zazu for their affection, and to the Quans for keeping a roof over my head. To Marilyn Bishara of Vixen Creations, and to all of the Vixen vixens: Gina, Laurel, Sue, Erica, Liz, and Liddy, Inka of Peartransmedia, Jade, Malia, Lara and Blade, and the bounty of bartering. To the entire *In Bed with Fairy Butch* staff for their steadfast assistance, especially Heidi, Tasha, Aimee and Kadijah, and to all of the *In Bed* patrons for their contributions to this book. To Yvette and Jane at Bagdad Cafe, Julie and Tim at Denny's, the boys at Jaguar, and my extended families in Dayton and Louisville. To Gretchen at *Curve* and the folks at *PlanetOut,* for spreading the word. To Ted for his company, and to Sparky and Brad Van Tine for their divine intervention. And finally to Kyra for providing me with an impetus toward health, peace, and balance and for her true love.

Contents

Illustrations

Introduction

Once you've reached adulthood, there just aren't many places left to play. Swing sets won't hold you, slides mess up your work clothes, and you're more likely to be running Excel on your computer than Sim City. Though the kids may have ejected you from the sandbox, sexuality is a playground available to you for the remainder of your days. By being playful with sex, you can try out new personas, genders, and power dynamics. You can travel to any time or place you like and make real personae divergent from your work-a-day life. You can share love and affection with a partner, explore new kinds of stimulation, make discoveries about yourself, and receive affirmation for secret parts of yourself. In other words, *sex is a wonderful chance to have fun*. I invite you to make strap-on sex—sex play using dildos and harnesses—a part of the festivities.

The first time I strapped it on I was six. I was playing house with some neighborhood kids, and being the major tomboy that I was, I insisted upon being The Dad. I took a rolled-up pair of socks and stuffed them into my tie-dyed Carter's (this was the early 70s) to approximate the bulge I knew dads had there. After being thoroughly chastised by my babysitter for this early attempt at gender-bending, I suppressed my strap-on exploits fully until age 21. At that time, an adventurous girlfriend and I went to town with a makeshift strap-on rig we devised from her father's boxers, some Levi's 501s, and a floppy ten-dollar, dead-on-arrival Caucasian dildo we named Andromeda (this was the mid-80s, and we thought we'd invented strap-ons.) My first store-bought strap-on rig was procured at a Los Angeles leather store when I was 23. It returned with me to my hometown of Dayton, Ohio. The first time I used it was in my mom and dad's house with a gal I had met at the local queer disco. Fortified by Popov vodka, we fell into my parents' bed and lost our official strap-on virginity together. (This was the late 80s and alcohol was a more common sexual lubricant than Astroglide.)

From these inauspicious beginnings, I started my career as a sex educator at the University of California, Berkeley in 1990, trained on the phone lines at San Francisco Sex Information, and then joined the Good Vibrations staff a year later. If you haven't heard of Good Vibrations, it is a resource with which you should become familiar. Joani Blank opened the first Good Vibrations store in 1977 in San Francisco to offer folks who wanted to buy sex toys and books a "clean, well-lighted" alternative to the typically sleazy adult bookstores, many of which offered inferior products, and were unwelcoming to women. Ten years later, a mail order operation was added to bring the Good Vibrations sales approach to people living outside of the Bay Area. Since then, the sex toy business has been revolutionized. Others have followed in the path Joani forged to create stores like Good Vibrations in many cities throughout North America and Europe. (Be sure to check out the Resources section at the back of the book to find out more about Good Vibrations and its sister stores.)

Back to my own strap-on sex pilgrimage. I'm a bigendered butch dyke. I came out as a lesbian in 1982 into Dayton, Ohio's small queer community, which dwelled mainly in the several bars and clubs available to us. If our sexual communication transpired in these dank surroundings, our sexuality itself was influenced by the vestiges of radical lesbian feminism which had trickled down from more urban centers. Dildos, particularly dildos harnessed to their user's pelvis, were taboo. As a matter of fact, in my circle penetration itself was regarded as no friend to lesbian sexuality. Though much of my own nascent adolescent and childhood masturbation had focused on inserting various objects inside myself to copious satisfaction, I learned that clitoral stimulation was much more enlightened, and well, *stimulating*. Since penetration had always been such a satisfying part of my sexual life, this proscription felt confusing and alienating to me in my fledging attempts to find my place in queer culture.

When I moved to San Francisco, the epicenter of the dyke sexual revolution of the late 80s, these prohibitions began to dissipate. I found lovers who were not only excited about penetration, but wanted to experiment with dildo and harness use as well. Through much trial and much error, I developed my skills as a strapper and began to explore how strap-on sex fit into the constellation of sexual power and gender dynamics I wanted to explore in my personal life. I threw myself into San

Francisco's rarefied sex culture, soaking up the copious sexual energy the city, with its public sex parties and leather street fairs, had to offer.

Indeed, I wasn't in Ohio anymore.

One of the most striking blows to my Midwestern sexual presumptions was my experience of heterosexual couples shopping for strap-ons—not just wild, tattooed and pierced, counterculture heterosexual people, though there were many of them, but the kind of heterosexual people I could have found among my parents' friends. I'll never forget the first such couple I helped at Good Vibrations. They were in their mid-50s, conservatively dressed, and since it was noon on Sunday, I assumed they had just come from church. I sauntered over, ready to show them to the massage oil and succulents section, when they asked to see the colors in which the Adam 4—an 8-inch long, $1\,7/8$-inch diameter dildo made by Scorpio Products—was available. They also wanted to pick the proper size Swashbuckler harness for the lady of the pair, and were hoping for a hue which matched her sweater dress ensemble. My life was changed.

As my career as a sex educator took hold, I soon began to offer workshops in strap-on sex, along with dyke sex workshops on oral, digital and anal sex, sex toys, sexuality and gender identity, and fisting. Dyke Sex Tips for Men and Dyke Sex Tips for Heterosexual Couples soon followed. In 1994, I began writing a sex advice column for *On Our Backs* magazine and developed a persona named Fairy Butch to do the talking for me. Fairy Butch is known to folks in the San Francisco Bay Area as the emcee of "In Bed with Fairy Butch," a twice-monthly erotic cabaret show. Fairy Butch's advice columns currently appear in *Curve* magazine, on PlanetOut (www.planetout.com), and on the Fairy Butch web site (www.fairybutch.com), as well as in a free email newsletter. (To sign up, email fb@fairybutch.com.) You'll find Fairy Butch's tips for strap-on sex throughout the book.

While you likely won't devote such an overwhelming portion of your life to sexuality, I encourage you to throw open those playground gates and immerse yourself in the fun and theater sex has to offer, and explore what strap-on sex in particular has to offer you. One caveat though: Please don't allow the information here to become a source of performance anxiety for you or your partner. Use this book rather as a jumping off place, a resource to help you fill your sexual toolbox. Expand on what I have written here, take what works for you, and leave the rest for a later time or for another person. And whether you've never seen a strap-on rig or you're an old pro looking for a few new tricks, I congratulate you for your bravery and sense of fun and adventure. I bid you happy strappin'!

San Francisco
May 2000

Myths About Strap-on Sex

1

There are many myths and misconceptions about strap-on sex and sex toy use. If you are confused about the role of strap-on dildos in your sex life, you're not alone. Here are some facts to allay your fears:

Sex toys are for couples with sexual problems.

This misconception has been created in part by the notorious misnomer, "marital aids," with which sex toys have often been saddled. The use of sex toys can be a great option for anyone—single or involved with one or more partners—who wants to expand their range of sexual possibilities. You may try sex toys to address a sexual difficulty, or you may simply want to elaborate on an already good thing. Some of the most sexually happy and healthy couples have sex toy collections which rival the wealth of King Tut's Dynasty.

Strap-on sex is only for lesbians.

Poppycock. Although hordes of lesbian and bisexual women proudly claim a strap-on rig or two among their valuables, many heterosexual men and women and gay men are proud members of the strap-on nation. A female member of a heterosexual couple can don a harness and dildo to penetrate her partner from behind, and a man can use a strap-on in conjunction with his erect or flaccid penis. The joys of dildos and harnesses are not limited to the Sapphic contingent.

Only impotent men use strap-on dildos.

Strap-on dildos can indeed enable men with erectile difficulties to penetrate their partners. But men may also strap them on to perform simultaneous vaginal and anal penetration, or to carry on after their erection is spent.

Men who want to be anally penetrated by a partner wearing strap-on dildo are really gay.

A butt's a butt and a prostate gland is a prostate gland, whether it belongs to a subscriber to *Playboy* or *Drummer*. Many heterosexual men love anal stimulation, while plenty of gay and bisexual men do not. Many heterosexual men long to surrender to a powerful female partner with a strap-on dildo, and some gay and bisexual men, especially those who equate anal receptivity with submission, won't let anyone near their asses. Body parts and particular sex acts are not the province of any particular gender or sexual orientation.

Lesbians who desire penetration really want to be with men.

Many lesbians enjoy vaginal and anal penetration with female fingers, tongues, or dildos. The vagina is rich with nerve endings, and many women enjoy vaginal—and especially G-spot—stimulation. In addition, the rhythmic motions of penetration can indirectly stimulate the clit- oris. Again, categories of sex acts, such as strap-on sex or anal penetration, are not specific to any one gender or sexual orientation.

A women who wears a dildo and harness suffers from penis envy or really wants to be a man.

While some female-bodied dildo-donners, such as female-to-male transsexuals (FTMs), do identify as men, the majority do not. Most female harness-wearers are happy to take off their strap-on rig and put it in the bureau drawer after sex. Some women revel in the fanta- sy of having a penis while they are wearing a dildo and harness. Other women are attracted to dildo and harness use less for the fantasy aspect than for the convenience and pleasure of strap-on sex.

Some FTMs enjoy their unaugmented genitalia just fine, whether or not they occasionally strap on a dildo. For those who want their genitals to appear more like the phalluses of biological males, there are a variety of options available. These include genital surgery and testosterone supplementation through cream, patches, or injections, all of which permanently increase the size of the clitoris. Genital surgery techniques include metoidaplasty, the surgical freeing of the testosterone- enlarged clitoris from the hood and surrounding tissue, and phalloplasty, the surgical construction of a full-sized penis created from skin and nerve grafts from other parts of the body. Other FTMs become adept at clit pumping, which temporarily increases the size of the clitoris.

The one who wears the dildo is in charge.

This is a very common misconception. Whether the phallus in question is a penis or a strap-on dildo, being the insertive partner does not necessarily mean you are in charge of the sex act. In many cases, the receptive partner may be running the show. She may enjoy telling you exactly when, where, and how to penetrate her ass or vagina. She may want you to remain perfectly still as she moves herself up and down to swallow the shaft of your toy. On the other hand, she may want to lie back and let you run the show. A variety of roles are available to either insertive or receptive partner. Good communication can help you figure out which roles will work in your play. Whether or not you are playing with power dynamics, the needs and limitations of the receptive partner must always define the parameters of strap-on play. Trustworthy insertive partners are aware of the health, safety, and pleasure of their partners.

Strap-on rigs are unattractive latex jobs complete with rubber panty and attached dildo, like those used in adult films.

Although there are a few decent, all-in-one strap-on models on the market, most of the dildos used in mainstream porn movies flop around like freshly caught rainbow trout in a canoe. Generally, your best bet is to select a dildo and a separate harness that best suit your needs. Although this approach requires more forethought than grabbing the first all-in-one combination you see at the local "dirty bookstore," it will yield far more satisfactory results in terms of both comfort and effectiveness.

Dildos and harnesses are available only at sleazy adult bookstores.

You don't have to visit a porn shop to buy a dildo. You'll find the best selection of sex toys—not to mention the best service and most comfortable atmosphere—in "clean, well-lighted" sex toy stores, such as San Francisco's Good Vibrations. Good Vibrations was established in

1977 with the idea that sex toys, supplies, books and videos should be available to all adults in a comfortable retail atmosphere, free from embarrassment, sleaze, and

---

Dear Fairy Butch,

I am a woman with a female partner. I'm concerned because my girlfriend really loves to be penetrated. She even wants me to fuck her with a dildo and harness. I know they're all in fashion, but doesn't her wanting something inside her vagina so badly really mean that she wants to be with a man?

—Worried in Wisconsin

Dear Worried:

Good Lord, Muffin, no. This is a variation of the "all men who want to be penetrated anally must really be gay" myth. Many queer girls have used this notion to terrorize themselves and their lovers. Just as many women who are attracted to men would rather have their partners focus on oral sex or other forms of sexual pleasuring besides penetration, innumerable lesbians adore having their vaginas and asses filled with female fingers, tongues, dildos. Many gay gals think it's grand to be fucked, and they want their female partners to do the fucking.

Just as there are straight men who long to feel their asses filled by a lover's fingers or strap-on, there are dykes who want to envelope a partner's strap-on dildo inside their cunt or ass. It's a mix-and-match proposition: you can be a woman-loving man and want it up the ass from your gal, or a full-fledged dyke and want to spread yourself for your gal's dick. Don't let anybody tell you different, Sister!

XOXOXOXO,

Fairy Butch

sexual harassment. Stores following this model have opened in several cities, including Toys in Babeland in Seattle and New York City, Grand Opening in Boston, A Woman's Touch in Madison, Wisconsin, and Womyn's Ware in Vancouver. Mail order businesses like Xandria and Blowfish cater to folks who do not live near sex toy stores which carry quality products or facilitate customer comfort. (See the Resources.)

Strap-on technique cannot be learned—either you are good at it, or you're not.

It's a mystery why folks think that sexual techniques—unlike riding a bicycle or swimming—cannot be learned. Perhaps it is because many people expect sex to be a mystical experience that "just happens." But knowing why a certain type of harness or lubricant will meet your needs, how to avoid poking your partner in the perineum, or how to last longer in the rear-entry position is neither mystical nor innate. You can acquire this information through fortuitous happenstance, through trial and error, or through books such as this one. You can become a more capable lover with education and practice.

If you are meant to wear a strap-on rig, you'll know it the first time you put it on; if you feel awkward, you're not meant to use it.

It's true that strap-on sex is not for everyone. But you may be feeling awkward because strap-on sex is not easy. There are very few experiences in life that are similar to strap-on sex, and there's no reason to think you'll do a flawless job the first time you try it. However, the more knowledge you gain and the more you practice, the more skillfully you will wield your strap-on rig.

Strap-on sex is unnatural.

What is natural? Is clothing natural? Indoor plumbing? Perfume? Linen bedding? None of these is any more natural than a dildo or harness, but I'll bet you wouldn't let that stand in the way of using them to enhance your life. Why should the notion of naturalness interfere with the use of a strap-on dildo if it brings you and your partner pleasure?

Anatomy: Learning the Lay of the Land

2

Do you harbor a hankering to be a strap-on stud? Perhaps your partner is the dildo-wearer, and you'd like to learn more about your role in strap-on sex. Whether you're the insertive or receptive partner, or interested in vaginal or anal penetration, learning more about sexual anatomy will help you enjoy strap-on sex.

Of course, written instruction is not a substitute for exploring your partner's body first-hand; very few women perfectly match a pelvic model, and not many men find their asses aptly represented by the line drawings of an anatomy textbook. Vaginal and rectal angles, lengths, and textures vary widely among individuals, and learning how your partner's canals are contoured—and how those contours change as she gets aroused and changes position—is one of the most important things to know for great strap-on sex. Explore your partner's vagina or anus with your fingers and hands first, particularly if you are with a new partner or you are new to strap-on sex. See "First-Hand Information" below.

The Front Door

The female urogenital system is a complex network of muscles, ligaments, blood vessels, glands, and erectile tissue, including the vagina, G-spot, clitoris, labia, perineum, and PC muscles. Knowing about the anatomy involved in vaginal penetration will help you learn how to best stimulate your partner—or yourself!

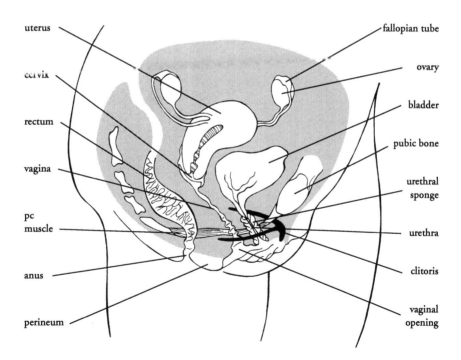

Illustration #1: Female anatomy

The Clitoris

The glans of the clitoris is the most sensitive part of the female genitals. It's situated beneath a thin, protective fold of tissue called the clitoral hood. The glans is dense with nerve endings and can be incredibly sensitive to touch. In fact, many women find direct stimulation of the glans to be excruciatingly intense, particularly if they are not sufficiently aroused.

The clitoral hood connects with the labia minora, or inner lips, surrounding the vaginal and urethral openings. The labia majora, which encircle the labia minora, are the thicker outer lips on which pubic hair grows. The labia minora are hairless and of the same texture as the mucous membranes of the vaginal opening.

Many people think the glans, which is the most visible portion of the clitoris, is the whole enchilada, but the glans is actually just the tip of the iceberg. The clitoral shaft, part of the internal structure of the clitoris, is a cord of tissue situated beneath the clitoral hood and attached to the suspensory ligament on the underside of the pubic bone. When a woman becomes aroused, her clitoral shaft becomes erect and engorges with blood; the suspensory ligament contracts and pulls the glans underneath the hood to protect it from over-stimulation. In this state, you can rub the clitoral hood lightly over the shaft and feel its hard, rod-shaped body, which feels like a flexible bit of cartilage. Many women enjoy this kind of indirect clitoral stimulation.

From its base, the clitoral shaft divides into two legs, called crura, which extend beneath the labia majora in a wishbone shape, one leg on either side of the vaginal opening. Each leg is approximately three inches in length and is independently attached to the ischium bones. When a woman is aroused, the crura become engorged with blood. Because the crura lie directly beneath the labia, they can be indirectly stimulated by tugging on the labia majora and labia minora, or through vaginal or anal penetration.

This understanding of internal female sexual anatomy offers a frame of reference for the myriad forms of pleasure women enjoy. Some women orgasm from direct stimulation of the clitoral glans or the G-spot; others prefer indirect stimulation of the clitoris, such as tugging on the labia minora, squeezing their legs together to create friction around the clitoris, or the pressure and thrusting of vaginal or anal penetration. Others love it all.

The dildo-wearer can also experience clitoral stimulation through strap-on sex. Thrusting into a partner and bumping against the partner's buttocks or pubic bone can stimulate the clitoris and is thus very pleasurable for many dildo strappers.

When I'm wearing my strap-on, I love fucking from behind, hard. The pounding gets me off.

The "balls" of the dildo provide my partner with indirect clitoral stimulation while she is fucking me.

The Vagina

The average vagina is about four inches in length, from the vaginal opening to the cervix at its end. The vaginal lining is composed of mucous membranes which are smooth in some places and roughly textured like a sponge in others. In its unaroused state, the walls of the vagina collapse in on one another, leaving just enough space for menstrual blood and other fluids to escape. The angle of the vagina varies from woman to woman. Learning how your partner's vagina is contoured, and how that contour changes as she becomes aroused and when she changes position, is one of the most important things you need to know to have great strap-on sex.

The deepest two-thirds of the vagina are sleek in texture, much like the inside surface of your mouth and cheeks. This part of the vagina is more sensitive to fullness and pressure than to other types of sensation. This means that a woman may not be able to tell when her cervix or the tissue deep inside her vagina has been scratched. She may be unaware that she has been injured by a rough-surfaced object during intercourse until the next day when she notices spotting. That's why it's so important to file your fingernails carefully before inserting your fingers into your partner's vagina, and to use only sex toys designed for penetration—those that are made of a pliable material and that are free of sharp edges or coarse surfaces. (If you have long fingernails, try stuffing cotton balls into the tips of a latex glove.)

The outer third of the vagina, closest to the opening, is rich in nerve endings and is more textured, with ridges and folds lining its surface. This part of the vagina can be very sensitive to touch, whether from fingers, dildos, or vibrators. The G-spot is located in the outer third of the vagina.

As a woman becomes sexually aroused, her vagina opens and her cervix retracts to the back of the vagina, making penetration easier and more pleasurable. The vagina begins to lubricate. The amount of lubrication a woman produces varies with the stage of her menstrual cycle, age, diet, level of arousal, recent sexual activity, and individual patterns. Although natural lubrication can go a long way in facilitating comfortable penetration, be sure to have a water-based lubricant available at all times.

The G-spot

The urethral sponge, or G-spot (named after gynecologist Ernst Grafenberg), is located two to three inches inside the vagina on the front wall of the vagina (closest to the hair-covered *mons pubis*). The G-spot is between the size of a dime and a half-dollar, and has a moist, spongy, rough texture. This spongy tissue is wrapped around the urethra (the tube carrying urine from the bladder) and protects it from injury during penetration. When a woman becomes aroused, the G-spot swells with fluid and pro-trudes a bit from the vaginal wall, making it easier to locate. The texture and sensitivity of the G-spot changes with increasing sexual excitement.

A few tips can help you find your partner's G-spot. Have your partner get on all fours with her back arched. Reach your fingers into her vagina with your palm facing downward, so that you can approach the G-spot with your sensitive fingertips rather than your fingernails. Another technique is to have your partner squat and bear down with her pubococcygeus (PC) muscles, the muscles of the pelvic floor. As she pushes out with her PC muscles, her G-spot will be pushed toward the vaginal opening and will be easier to reach. This technique is particularly helpful for people with short fingers.

While many women relish direct G-spot stimulation, others find it irritating, especially if they are not suffi-ciently aroused. Ask your partner if this is the case for her; if so, start with indirect stimulation of her G-spot, increas-ing the intensity as her arousal mounts.

Since the G-spot surrounds the urethra and is adja-cent to the bladder, many women feel an urge to urinate when this spot is touched, especially if too much stimula-tion is given too soon. Your partner may be able to avoid this sensation by emptying her bladder before sex. You can reassure her by placing a towel underneath her before penetration.

With intense G-spot stimulation, some women ejac-ulate fluid through the urethra from the vulvovaginal

Dear Fairy Butch,

    Is it still possible for a girl such as myself to find her G-spot? I've been looking for it forever, but end up feeling like I have to pee! Help!

                           —Holding It in Hawaii

Dearest Holding,

    Stop in the name of love!

    Stop holding it in, Sugar. When a gal's G-spot is first stimulated, she often feels as though she has to pee like a racehorse! But never fear, it is not the specter of urinary incontinence that has been raised, but rather the initial stirrings of your urethral sponge, or G-spot.

    Now, nobody says that you have to become a G-spot aficionado. But if that is indeed your aim, here's what you do. First of all, go pee. Second, put a towel underneath your hind end. These precautions will reassure you that you don't actually have to pee whilst spot spelunking, and that if you do ejaculate, you can go with the flow. Get yourself in a comfy position, perhaps with your ankles behind your ears or on all fours, and find that juicy little brain hemisphere located on the anterior wall of your vagina. Experiment with light and firm touches; you might well feel like you have to pee, but remember that there is no urine left to release.

    With that knowledge in mind, push past that peeing impulse and keep on stroking. You are likely to find that the urge to pee has been replaced by urges of a different nature entirely. Give it a whirl, little pearl!

XOXOXOXOXO,

Fairy Butch

glands, the small vessels on either side of the vagina. Contrary to a popular fallacy, this fluid is not urine, despite the fact that there is often a lot of it and it may be expelled with great force. The fluid is actually similar in composition to a man's semen without the sperm.

The Urethra

If you are under the impression that a woman urinates from her vagina, you are far from alone in this popular misconception. Urine actually flows from the bladder through the urethral opening, located just above the entrance to the vagina and below the clitoris. Many women find direct stimulation of the urethral opening irritating. Be careful not to introduce bacteria into the urethra, since doing so may lead to infection. You can lessen the risk of urinary tract infections by peeing after penetrative sex, washing hands and sex toys, and using fresh latex gloves and condoms with each new partner or sexual activity.

The Perineum, Pubic Bone, and PC Muscles

The perineum is an area of muscular tissue between the anus and the vagina in women, and between the anus and the base of the scrotum in men. Accidentally poking a dildo into the perineum can be painful, and must be considered when adopting an angle at which to brandish your strap-on dildo. Conversely, massaging the perineum, by applying gentle but firm pressure directly or through the walls of either the vagina or the rectum, can be an excellent way to relax your partner in preparation for strap-on play.

The flange (or base) of the dildo in a harness rests against the public bone. If you don't have much subcutaneous fat covering your pubic bone, you may want to choose a harness that has a flap of leather between the flange and the pubis, or put a bit of soft cloth between your pubic mound and the flange of the dildo The pubo-coccygeus (PC) muscles girdle the pelvic floor in a figure-eight formation from the pubic bone to the tailbone in both men and women. These muscles are the ones used to stop the flow of urine in midstream. The PC muscles contract during orgasm, and learning how to strengthen and relax them can greatly enhance sexual pleasure and control.

The Back Door

Ah, the ass—abundant potential, so often uncultivated! While anal exploits aren't for everyone, more people yearn to open the back door than actually come a-knock-ing. Part of the reason behind this unrequited fancy are the taboos associated with anal sex. Also, because the anus is a conduit for elimination of feces, anal sex is thought by some to be unclean. Anal exploration through strap-on sex is an erotic possibility open to everyone—men and women. Anal anatomy includes the anus, exter-nal and internal sphincter muscles, anal canal, rectum, and perineum.

The anus is the external opening to the rectum. It is encircled by two muscles, the external and internal sphincters. While the internal sphincter is controlled by the autonomic nervous system and thus responds sponta-neously to stimulation, the external sphincter can be relaxed and tensed voluntarily. Just as the muscles in your neck or back may become constricted with the day's ten-sion or in response to particular emotions, so may the external sphincter. If you pay attention, you can feel your external sphincter relax along with the rest of your body as you take a hot bath, receive a massage, or engage in some other activity to reduce tension.

The anal canal extends from the anus at its opening, through the rectum, to the sigmoid colon in a loose "S" shape. Several inches in, the anal canal curves toward the public bone. The rectum initially follows the lead of the anal canal, first turning toward the pubic bone, then bending back toward the tailbone as the body of the organ unfolds. The tailbone is located directly behind the rectum; take care not to contradict the curvature of the rectum during penetration, since compressing the soft anorectal tissue against the hard surface of the tailbone can be quite painful.

It is very important to explore the curve of your partner's anal canal and rectum carefully with your fingers before engaging in strap-on sex. Not only does each ass possess its own idiosyncrasies, but the size and touch of your fingers can provide a warm-up for dildo penetration.

The anus is rich with nerve endings and is very responsive to the level of trust, comfort, and arousal the receptive partner feels, as well as to the conditioned response he or she has developed during previous anal sex experiences.

Anorectal anatomy is fragile in comparison to the vagina, which has copious natural lubrication and thicker layers of mucous membrane. The rectum is lined with a thin layer of mucous membrane and produces very little natural lubrication. Needless to say, it is important to keep plenty of lubricant on hand for safe and pleasurable anal fun.

The Prostate Gland

The prostate gland is a walnut-shaped organ that produces ejaculatory fluid in men. It is located about three inches inside the anus, behind the pubic bone and below the bladder, and can be reached through the wall of the rectum. Many men enjoy stimulation of the prostate, either alone or in addition to genital stimulation. The prostate is homologous to a woman's G-spot, and similarly, many men prefer indirect stimulation of the anus and rectum to direct stimulation of the prostate. Some men may desire more intense prostate stimulation only after becoming sufficiently aroused through general body stimulation or stimulation of the cock and balls.

All I have to say is that men who don't make friends with their prostates are missing out on some good fun. Anal penetration has given me the most mind-blowing, body-shaking experiences I have ever had, alone or partnered.

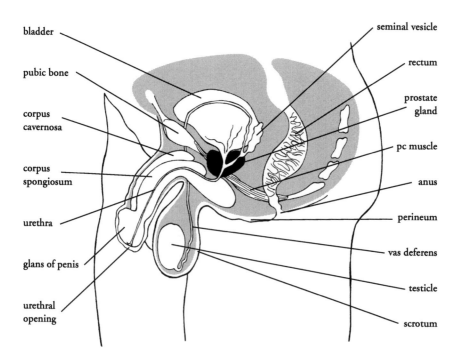

Illustration #2: Male anatomy

First-Hand Information

Nothing can match the intelligence of your fingers as they learn the angle of your female partner's vagina, the thickness of her perineum, or the depth at which you encounter a male partner's prostate gland. If you allow yourself time to explore your partner's body, the information you gather will help you wield your dildo to its fullest potential.

Set aside an hour or two to explore your partner's body—a fact-finding mission, if you will. Allow this time for gathering information rather than the pursuit of orgasm, though you needn't be deterred if your research should lead to such a happy consequence. This exercise is best done in the spirit of fun and education, free from performance pressure.

Begin by discussing which areas and activities you will investigate and which are off limits. If you intend to switch roles, decide which of you will start out as the insertive partner and which will start out as the receptive partner. Focus on one partner at a time. Set up a space in which you both feel comfortable and warm, and be sure that there are ample pillows, plenty of water nearby, and sufficient light. Free yourself from any possible distractions and interruptions. If you like, light some candles, burn some incense, and play some relaxing music. Make sure that you've got plenty of water-based lubricant and latex gloves.

You may wish to play naughty nurse or doctor-and-patient to lighten the mood. Or the insertive partner can blindfold her mate to help both partners feel less self-conscious. In any case, what matters is that the insertive partner feel free to gather information and the receptive partner feel comfortable with the investigation.

Dear Fairy Butch,

My girlfriend and I have recently discovered the joys of anal sex, and one of the things that really drives her insane is to be penetrated in the ass and the pussy at the same time. My question is one of logistics: I want to be able to kiss and touch her during the process. We've tried using a small dildo in her ass while I fuck her pussy, but before long, it gets pushed out in all the excitement. I feel like I need a third hand. Any suggestions?

—Octopus Wannabe

Dear Puss:

Darling—you don't need a third hand, you need a butt plug! Butt plugs are marvelous, cupcake, and are designed for just such an occasion. Narrow at the top and wider toward the middle, *le plug* becomes markedly narrow again, and ends with a flange which prevents the toy from escaping up your tush. What makes this toy different from other toys (the rarely asked fifth Passover seder question) is that it stays put—hands free! You see, the sphincter muscle opens up around the bulbous part of the plug, and then clasps around the narrow recess. This makes it ideal for use while simultaneously fucking or eating pussy, making out, breast fondling, riding the bus, visiting with the in-laws, or writing a sex advice column, for that matter. They are available in a variety of materials, but I hold a particular fondness for silicone, as it can be disinfected when the party's over. Have fun with the extra digits, girlfriend!

XOXOXOXO,

Fairy Butch

Begin with whole body and face massage, and progress from general to specific stimulation, from the chest and nipples to the buttocks and inner thighs, and then toward the genitals and anus. Move gradually, allowing your partner to become increasingly comfortable with opening his or her body to you. As you progress in massaging your partner, you will increase the flow of blood to each area you touch, and thereby enhance your partner's sexual arousal.

After your partner is sufficiently aroused and has indicated that she or he is ready, use your fingers to explore your partner's vagina or anus. Note the texture of the G-spot, the location of the cervix, or the curve of the rectum. You can use a plastic speculum and small flashlight for vaginal exploration. Get verbal feedback from your partner—ask what feels good and what not-so-good. You might want to employ a technique used by sex researchers Masters and Johnson that involves gradually changing the way you touch your partner. Your partner assigns a number between - 3 and + 3 to indicate his or her level of pleasure or displeasure: -3 for very unpleasant, -2 for somewhat unpleasant, -1 for mildly unpleasant, 0 for neutral, +1 for mildly pleasant, +2 for very pleasant, and +3 for extremely arousing. Using this method, you can get very specific feedback as you experiment with different types of touches.

Consider the way your partner's genital structures look, and particularly how they feel in various stages of arousal. Note the way your partner's vagina or rectum is curved. Ask your partner to change position; experiment with raising his legs as you examine him internally, put a pillow underneath her hips, or have him turn around on all fours. Pay careful attention to the ways in which the internal curve changes with your partner's movements. Observe which positions provide easiest access to a male partner's prostate gland or a female partner's G-spot and cervix.

Once you are familiar with sexual anatomy in general and your partner's body in particular, you will be far more confident in your ability to provide the kind of stimulation he or she desires.

Dildos: The Long and the Short of It

3

If you visited the dildo section of a woman-owned sex toy store 15 years ago, you might have thought you'd happened upon a Midwestern farm. There among the vibrators and lubricants, you would be sure to have found dildos in the shape of zucchini, bananas, corncobs, dolphins, cats, birds, and other carbon-based life forms. This Disco-era whimsy was augmented by silicone toys in the shape of fingers, fists, and praying women. These aesthetics were frequently seized upon by pro-sex feminists eager to reclaim the pleasures of penetrative sex, but without the phallic imagery they found objectionable. Now you'll have better luck tracking down your ocean mammals at Sea World and your produce at the local Farmer's Market—the tide has turned in dildo production and has brought with it toys that bear a closer resemblance to penises than porpoises.

You may still spy the occasional bluebird looking over your shoulder from the top shelf at Toys in Babeland or Grand Opening, but dildo designs of late vary less in shape than in color. Most dildo styles are either the wavy, nondescript "Jane Does" or the phallic-looking realistic models favored by those who wish to incorporate gender play into their strap-on use. Dildos now come in a veritable rainbow of colors for those who fancy a package with a bit of panache. Don't be shocked to find an otherwise realistic dick in bright fuchsia or candy corn stripes of yellow and orange—in some circles, such hues are much preferred to their "skin-toned" shelf mates.

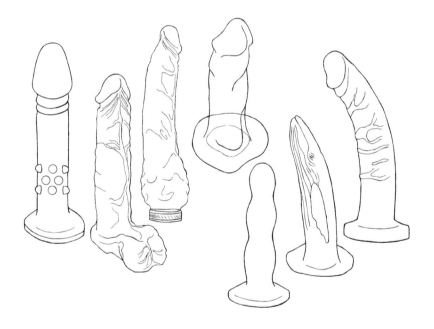

Illustration #3: Dildos

Before we got our newest dildos, I thought I'd only like the skin-colored ones. Now, I appreciate the different colors because they somehow allow for greater ownership of the dick as a butch cock.

I have a really hard time with representational toys. That is, those with veins, skin color, and anatomically accurate parts. I prefer less realism. My current favorites are a long, silver, glittery dildo, and a thicker, ripply, black "Jane Doe" model. I'm both a size queen and a fashion queen, so glitter, glamour, and size are all impor-tant to me.

Material Girls (and Boys)

Historically, dildos have been carved from a variety of materials, both prosaic and precious. These have included wood, steel, ivory, and marble. The purposes of most contemporary strappers, however, will best be served by toys made from pliant materials such as sili-cone, polyvinylchloride (PVC), thermal plastic (Cyber-skin), latex, soft plastic, and "mystery rubber"—my catch-all label for the rest of the synthetic rubber used in dildos. Though your local sex toy emporium may sell dildos made from harder materials such as metal, glass, wood, or hard plastic, these are not well-suited for strap-on sex.

Silicone

Silicone is widely regarded by sex toy aficionados as the *crème de la crème* of dildo materials. It is characterized by a tight molecular structure that renders dildos highly conducive to body heat and vibration. (Try soaking a sili-cone dildo in warm water prior to use for a pleasantly toasty surface.) Silicone repels dirt and bacteria, and does not fall apart with extended friction. Although several larger sex toy manufacturers have begun to mass produce such toys, most silicone dildos are still made by small women-owned companies, such as Vixen Creations, Scorpio, and Dills for Does. Craftspeople in these studios mold each toy by hand in a wide variety of sizes, styles, and colors, including swirl patterns, glamour shades such as silver and gold glitter, and clever glow-in-the-dark models. Just picture the visual spectacle you can create in a dark room as your dildo slips in and out of your partner's ass.

Because sexually transmitted diseases and bacterial infections can be spread through the use of shared sex toys, silicone is the natural choice for those who want to share their toys or switch between anal and vaginal penetration. Anal bacteria should never be introduced into the vagina, even the anal bacteria and vagina of the same woman. Silicone can be fully disinfected rather than merely cleaned. Simply place the toy in a pan of boiling water for three minutes, and it will be rendered safe for any orifice—yours or that of a friend. Silicone can also be fully disinfected by wiping it with bleach or throwing it into the top rack of your dishwasher. This level of sterilization cannot be achieved with toys made from other materials; use condoms to avoid bacterial infections and sexually-transmitted diseases. Even though silicone can be thoroughly disinfected, condoms are still useful when things get hot and heavy and you want to move quickly from one sexual activity to another.

Because each silicone toy is carefully manufactured and inspected by hand, and because the material is so durable and hygienic, such toys are superior in many ways to those that are machine-produced using cheaper materials. Unlike some other types of dildos, silicone toys will not as quickly reveal the ravages of time. With proper care, silicone dildos can maintain their rigidity for many years. Although a $70 silicone toy may seem expensive, with regular use you will come to appreciate its value. I have several silicone dildos I bought a decade ago that are still in pristine shape, while rubber toys I purchased at the same time have long since bit the dust.

Miracle substance status notwithstanding, there are a few disadvantages to silicone toys. First, the major drawback of silicone toys is their cost. Because silicone is expensive, the price of each toy is dependent upon the amount of the material used to create it, much to the chagrin of size queens. The price goes up as well with the added expense of incorporating special materials such as

---

Dear Fairy Butch,

Hey there, sex toy queen, what's up with those new jewel-colored dildos that are all the rage these days? What is that stuff exactly?

—Would-Be Jeweled Jezebel

Dear Jez:

Scads of multi-colored, diaphanous dildos have made their way onto the sex toy world stage of late, and if their appearance has left you bewildered, be baffled no more—it's PVC. That's right, those tantalizing jelly toys in sapphire, ruby, and emerald are made from PVC, the same stuff used to make children's toys and many household items—and even fetish wear!

XOXOXOXO,

Fairy Butch

glitter or creating bi-colored swirl effects. Expect to pay from $30 to $90 for a silicone dildo.

Second, there are very few hyper-realistic silicone dildos from which to choose. If you're going for manly realism—bluish veins, pinkish glans, and convincing skin texture—you'll find a dramatically wider selection among the mystery rubber dildos, including those modeled after the penises of porn legends such as Jeff Stryker and Sean Michaels.

A third factor to consider when purchasing a silicone toy is its fragility in the face of sharp objects. Once a tear has been made in the surface of a silicone toy, you can pretty much write it off. Keep your silicone dildo out of the reach of Fluffy's paws, and when traveling, wrap it in a thick sock inside your suitcase. Finally, silicone dildos should not be used with silicone lubricants because the solvent in the lubricant (which keeps the silicone liquid) can cause the toys to disintegrate.

PVC

Many multicolored, diaphanous dildos have made their way onto sex toy shelves. These tantalizing jelly toys in hues of sapphire, ruby, and emerald are made from polyvinylchloride (PVC), the same material used to make pipes, door frames, children's toys, and fetish clothing.

Sex toys manufactured from PVC are machine-made and mass-produced. These dildos are quite inexpensive—usually in the $15 to $50 range—sturdy, smooth, and often translucent. They come in a dazzling array of bright colors ranging from the jewel variety to those that more closely resemble Orange Crush with carbonation bubbles.

PVC is a plastic, but it has a pleasantly smooth, rubbery feel. It is denser than most synthetic rubbers, yet not nearly as impenetrable as silicone, so it can abrade with friction and cannot be disinfected. You will often see visible pores on the surface of PVC toys—a good reason to adorn your PVC dildos with condoms, especially if you intend to share them or use them for both vaginal and anal penetration. PVC toys should be cleaned frequently with an antibacterial product such as ForPlay Adult Toy Cleanser or Hibiclens, and stored in a cloth sack or a thick cotton sock.

Solid PVC dildos have a considerable heft to them. If your PVC toy is sufficiently supported by your harness, its weight may be a boon to serious pounding. On the other hand, large PVC dildos suspended by an inadequate harness may droop. Their heavy weight makes these toys great for robust, hand-held penetration, provided you have the arm strength to go the duration. PVC is a good material for vibrating toys, including those designed with a flared base or flange and an external remote control unit. These toys are priced in the $20 to $40 range, and are an inexpensive way to combine the pleasures of vibration and strap-on sex.

Cyberskin

Cyberskin, the product name for dildos made from thermal plastic (a mixture of PVC and silicone), is the latest contender for your dildo dollar. Sex toy consumers are abuzz about these toys because dildos made from this material feel so much like, well, *dicks*. Cyberskin toys are manufactured using a sophisticated injection-molding machine—originally designed by NASA engineers—that is able to precisely vary the density of the plastic throughout the toy. This allows for dildos that feel rigid like erectile tissue toward the center, but supple and malleable like skin at the surface.

Cyberskin is also used to make sheaths designed to fit over vibrators, dildos, and even penises. They roll on like a condom, but can be reused again and again with proper cleaning. Unlike condoms, however, Cyberskin sheaths are not a sufficient means of safer sex or birth control. The high molecular density of Cyberskin makes it flexible and resilient, endowing it with a "material memory" that allows it to recover its original form after being tugged, stroked, or sucked.

The manufacturer has patented both the material and the unique, realistic feel of these toys under the name Virtual Touch. Cyberskin dildos, some of which are equipped with vibrators, range in price from $25 to $80. While these toys may feel like the real deal, their luminescent monochromatic coloring bears closer resemblance to the member of an extraterrestrial than that of a human being. Those seeking a more realistic-looking dildo may be better served by a synthetic rubber model.

Thermal plastic is a magnet for dirt and dust, and keeping these toys sanitary can be quite a process, so protect your Cyberskin toys with condoms. Clean them with warm water and an antibacterial soap such as Hibiclens or with ForPlay Adult Toy Cleanser, and rinse them thoroughly. Cyberskin should not be boiled and cannot be disinfected. Pat your toy dry with a cloth towel, since tissue will adhere like crazy to Cyberskin. Dust the dildo with cornstarch to keep it fresh until your next use. Cornstarch will prevent lint and dirt from sticking to the surface; do not use talcum powder to dust your toys, as some studies have linked the use of talc to cervical cancer. Store your Cyberskin toy in a cool, dry place in a toy sack or a thick cotton sock. When you're ready to use it again, simply wash off the cornstarch or roll on a condom. Avoid using silicone lubricant with Cyberskin dildos because the silicone in the lube can cause these toys to disintegrate.

Latex

Latex has become a catch-all category for many sex toys—even those that don't contain latex at all. Actual latex dildos are most often black, and their surface is characterized by a dull, almost dusty quality. Manufacturers will often wrap a sheet of latex around a stiffer material, such as compressed foam, to lend firmness to the finished product. If the flared base of a latex dildo is also made of latex, it will likely be quite floppy and thus not ideal for strap-on use. If this is the case, you can use a donut-shaped SlipNot accessory to reinforce the flange so that it is rigid enough to use with a harness. The SlipNot will also prevent the base from slipping through the opening of the harness.

Latex has a fairly loose molecular structure that oxidizes over time, and dildos made from this material may break down with use. You can extend their life by storing them in a cool, dry place, away from sunlight. Oil-based lubricants should never be used with latex, as petroleum disintegrates the material on contact; use only water-based lubricants with these toys. Like PVC, latex can be cleaned but not disinfected, so condom use is recommended. To clean latex toys, brush gently with a soft-bristle food scrubber, warm water, and an antibacterial product such as ForPlay Adult Toy Cleanser or Hibiclens.

Latex dildos range in price from $30 to $60.

Soft Plastic

Soft plastic dildos are very inexpensive and have a waxy, moderately pliant surface. There are a wide variety of toys made from this material priced under $20, many of which are equipped with vibrators. Make sure that the model you choose has a base wide enough to use in a harness. Soft plastic dildos appear most frequently in a pinkish color that many toy salespeople have dubbed DOA Caucasian, although a few manufacturers have broadened the racial representation of their product lines. Others have added colors that do not attempt to approximate human skin tones, such as lavender and turquoise.

The process by which soft plastic toys are manufactured is similar to that of latex toys. Often a layer of plastic is molded over a stiff foam core, so that the toys can stand up to use. Like other non-silicone dildos, soft plastic toys attract dirt, dust, and bacteria. They cannot be disinfected, and stains are difficult to remove. These toys should be used with condoms, cleaned well, and stored in a toy sack or a thick sock in a dark, dry place.

Mystery Rubber

For our purposes, let's use the term *mystery rubber* for the remainder of the many synthetic rubber dildos you may encounter, each composed of any one of several different synthetic ingredients. If you have visited a porn shop, you have no doubt seen "dongs" of all shapes and sizes fashioned from this material. These toys are machine-pressed, assembly-line products marketed as "novelty items" by such manufacturers as Doc Johnson and Swedish Erotica. They are most often peach-colored, but occasionally brown. Usually they are displayed mounted on blisterboard under transparent plastic, so you cannot handle them in the store. These dildos are sold in tens of thousands of outlets throughout the globe and on the Internet.

Ease of purchase is one of several benefits afforded by mystery rubber. Mystery rubber dildos come in a wide range of prices (from $10 to $100), with a variety of options under $25. Their affordability makes them good starter toys for those who are not yet ready to fully commit to an expensive purchase, and good sizing tools for those who are ready for an upgrade. There is an excellent selection of highly realistic mystery rubber dildos—no doubt your favorite male porn star has had his likeness carved from synthetic rubber, perhaps equipped with a suction cup to attach to your shower wall or refrigerator door. Mystery rubber toys tend to be more flexible than other dildos, which can be a boon to double dildo users. This feature can be a disadvantage in strap-on sex, however, because synthetic rubber often loses its rigidity and becomes floppy over time. This can be truly frustrating since you want your dildo to move in tandem with the motions of your hips in strap-on sex.

Another drawback of mystery rubber is its porousness. Because its molecules are loosely bound, it easily attracts dirt and bacteria, and it holds the grime and

Decorative Dildos

Although many people enjoy dildos made from unyielding materials such as hard plastic, wood, metal, or glass for penetration by hand—and while they may serve as intriguing objets d'art—they are not designed for strap-on sex.

Your favorite clear Lucite dildo may well prove delightful for solo play, but even experienced strappers should refrain from using such a toy with a harness. Just imagine the havoc a hard plastic base could wreak on the public bone of a lass whose partner's endorphin rush has propelled her toward overzealous thrusting. As for the use of glass in the saddle, as it were, the mind boggles at the dangers such a choice could pose for both insertive and receptive partners. Save these beauties for penetration by hand—or for adorning your coffee table.

germs within its large pores. The surface of synthetic rubber toys abrade easily with friction. Like pencil erasers, if you rub them firmly, you'll see little bits of worn off rubber collect in your hand. Imagine the same thing happening inside your vagina or anus. Synthetic rubber also attracts pigments, making it difficult to remove stains.

Because mystery rubber toys cannot be disinfected, use them with condoms, especially if you share your toys. Always use condoms for anal play with these dildos to avoid introducing anal flora into the vagina. You may even want to consider buying separate toys for anal use. Clean synthetic rubber toys after each use with an antibacterial cleaning product such as Hibiclens or ForPlay Adult Toy Cleanser, and store them in a toy sack away from light, moisture, and heat. Even with these precautions, don't expect a synthetic rubber dildo to be a legacy item in your trousseau.

Size Matters

Many times in my years as a dildo salesperson, a customer has presented me with his or her partner and asked, "Which size dildo should we buy?"—as if I could tell by the fit of his Levi's. You can bet that I won't be able to judge a good fit for your boyfriend's butt just by looking at him. Nonetheless, many people who are interested in trying strap-on sex select a dildo in just this manner—trying to match the size of the toy to the size of the body into which it will be inserted. This method is a mistake. I have met many a diminutive lass who begged for more when filled with a two-inch-diameter dildo or fist, and legions of sturdy boys who blanch at the notion of taking more than a one-inch model between their cheeks. Questions of size, however, can be easy to resolve on your own if you are willing to invest a bit of time.

Let's begin with a quick primer on measurements. Dildo size is based on two factors, length and width. Width is determined by either of two measures: circumference which is the distance around the dildo, or diameter, which is the width of a cross-section of the toy. Diameter is used far more frequently for sizing dildos; since you can't very well cut up each toy you'd like to assess, you must rely on information provided by the manufacturer. Dildo diameter typically ranges from 1 to 2 $\frac{1}{2}$ inches. Although the difference in these dimensions may seem minute, it is, in fact, the difference between a finger and a forearm. When in doubt, err toward the more slender dildo—if it turns out to be too small, you can use the toy for anal play or as a warm-up for a subsequent, larger purchase.

Length is another matter entirely. For strap-on sex, you will want a dildo long enough to allow for powerful thrusting. If you are unsure which length to purchase, your appraisal process should be the opposite of that used for diameter—pick the longer toy. Why? You will need to factor in an extra $\frac{3}{4}$ to 1 inch for the thickness of the harness; allow for the loss of even more length when adding other toys or a SlipNot to the arrangement. A protruding belly may be a consideration in choosing toy length. If the dildo is too long, the insertive partner can abbreviate the depth of her thrusts. On the other hand, if the dildo is too short, the range of motion is limited.

This is not to say that there is one perfectly sized dildo for each person, like a shoe size. A receptive partner may prefer different toys at different times, and her tastes may be influenced by a variety of factors including changes related to pregnancy and childbirth, age, and phase of the menstrual cycle. During ovulation and menstruation, for example, some women may prefer a larger dildo. Likewise, a 7-inch long by 1 $\frac{5}{8}$ inch thick toy that was a challenge for a woman prior to pregnancy may be her warm-up toy after she has given birth.

Another factor that may influence size preference is conditioned response, the process by which the body becomes acclimated to stimulus and then responds more quickly and fully. An experienced receptive partner will likely enjoy a larger toy than he or she did the first time out. Similarly, a person who enjoys being penetrated frequently will likely be able to accommodate a larger toy than one who is penetrated only occasionally. Size preferences can vary even within the same act; a receptive partner may wish to start out with a smaller toy and switch to something larger as she becomes more aroused. Finally, partners may choose dildo size based on the kind of sex they desire. To wit, a receptive partner who finds a 1 $\frac{1}{2}$ inch diameter toy perfect for a languorous, leisurely love fest may hanker for a 2-incher when the action heats up.

> The first dildo I ever saw was a Jeff Stryker. I wondered if it would cause an earache. It didn't.

Harnesses: Bound for Glory

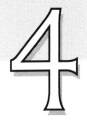

Dildo harnesses are marvelous devices designed to secure a dildo to the body of the wearer to enable her to penetrate a partner. Although harnesses come in a wide array of styles, all consist of straps which secure the garment to the wearer and some means by which a dildo (or other toy) is fastened to the harness itself. They have been used in many cultures and across an impressive expanse of history. They were depicted on the feet and hands of ambitious male suitors in the sexual tomes of ancient Japan, warned against in the legal proclamations of medieval Europe, and considered *de rigeur* for mid-20th century butch dykes in the United States.

Why use a harness? Why not just pick up your toy and hammer it home? Some people appreciate dildo harnesses for their utilitarianism. With a harness, you can penetrate a partner while keeping your hands free for other kinds of stimulation. For example, you may use a harness because it allows you to penetrate your partner from behind while at the same time caressing her breasts and tugging at her nipples. Perhaps you appreciate how easily you can receive vaginal or anal stimulation yourself while penetrating a partner, through the use of a harness cuff designed to hold a dildo inside the insertive partner. As a man, you might harness a dildo above your flaccid penis to penetrate a partner when you do not have an erection.

> I like to wear a harness because of the freedom it allows my hands and mouth. I also like to wear a harness because it makes me feel like an animal.

Other harness users are drawn to strap-on sex for the skin-on-skin intimacy it permits. The possibilities for sexual embrace during strap-on sex are endless. As the receptive partner in missionary position sex, for example, you can wrap your legs around your partner's torso and push upward while you kiss or look into each other's eyes. As the insertive partner in rear-entry sex, you can wrap your arms around your partner's hips and back. In the side-by-side position, you can maintain full-body contact in a gentle, languorous fashion.

Finally, many harness users appreciate the gender play possibilities of strap-on sex. Perhaps you enjoy the appearance of an erect dick suspended between your legs or bobbing from your partner's pelvis. Among those who appreciate the gender significance of strap-on sex, you may find female-to-male transsexuals (FTMs), butch dykes, feminine women who love the genderfuck of combining a big dick with lace garter belts and stockings, and men who relish the spectacle of a second erect phallus jutting out in tandem with their own erect penis.

Harness Styles

Harnesses can be classified into three basic styles:
• thong-style or two-strap harnesses
• jockstrap-style or three-strap harnesses
• miscellaneous style harnesses, including thigh harnesses
  and harnesses that attach a dildo to furniture.

Thong-style harnesses have a center strap which travels between the wearer's legs from crotch to buttocks. The center strap attaches to the front panel of the garment and to the strap that circles the wearer's waist. Thong-style harnesses come in a wide variety of models. At the ascetic end of the spectrum are models such as the basic triangle harness, which uses a rubber O-ring within a triangle of leather to hold the dildo against the wearer's pubic mound. If you want something a bit fancier, you can opt for a deluxe model such as the Swashbuckler or the Tuxedo Double, which include a cuff hold a dildo or butt plug inside the vagina or anus of the wearer. Both feature a thick, adjustable center strap attached to a metal O-ring.

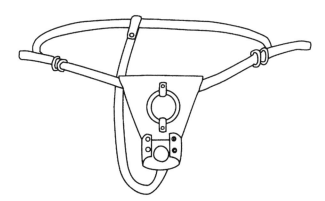

Illustration 4: Stormy Leather® Tuxedo Double Harness

Jockstrap-style harnesses are similar to their name-sake, with a belt that goes around the wearer's waist and two straps that encircle the thighs and attach to the back of the belt. This style leaves the vagina and anus accessible. Jockstrap-style harnesses are preferred by people who dislike the feel of a strap through their crotch and between their buttocks. As with thong-style harnesses, jockstrap-style harnesses range from simpler models, such as the Texas Two Strap, to deluxe versions such as the Jewel Buckling and the Terra Firma. The Texas Two Strap secures a dildo against the wearer's pubic mound by means of a rubber O-ring embedded in the front panel of the harness. The leg straps swing around each thigh and attach to D-rings hanging from either side of the waist belt. The Jewel Buckling and Terra Firma harnesses incorporate a leather flap behind the harness' O-ring that can be positioned behind the flange of a dildo to protect the wearer from discomfort of the base of the dildo pulling on the pubic hair or jutting into the flesh. This model uses buckles rather than D-rings for a more secure fit. The leg straps can be adjusted around the harness wearer's balls—whether they are synthetic or flesh—for greater comfort.

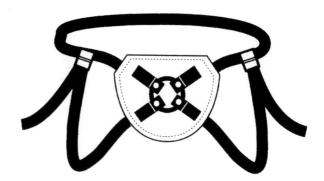

Illustration #5: Stormy Leather® Malibu Terra Firma Harness

Our harness is jockstrap style harness. It moves with my boyfriend and doesn't slip. It allows for a more natural and fluid feel for both of us.

How to Put on a Thong or Jock Harness

To put on a harness, first place the dildo through the O-ring. Loosely fasten the strap on one side and place your foot through the fastened strap. After stepping into the harness, fasten the other side and adjust the straps to achieve a secure fit. Tighten the harness evenly on each side of your body to a snug but comfortable fit. If there is a significant amount of excess strap length after you have adjusted your rig (and you don't expect to gain much weight), cut the excess evenly off each side of your harness, leaving enough slack so that the straps can still be pulled easily through the D-rings or buckles. Light a match and carefully singe the ends of the cut straps to prevent fraying.

When selecting a harness to wear around your midsection, it is a good idea to try on both thong and jock styles to determine which works best for your body. Some people like the way a thong-style harness holds a dildo firmly against their body, while others prefer a jockstrap-style harness. The decision is fairly subjective, and depends to a large extent on how your body weight is distributed. A friend and I once argued the merits of thong-style versus jockstrap-style harnesses, with each of us vehemently contending that her preferred style positioned the dildo at a more fortuitous angle. It finally dawned on us that our vastly different body types were likely a major factor in our divergent preferences.

Not all harnesses strap to the wearer's midsection at all—in fact, some don't even strap to the strapper! The miscellaneous category consists of thigh harnesses and models that strap dildos onto objects rather than people. These harnesses are generally of a more simple design than either thong-style or jockstrap-style models. Most consist of an O-ring secured inside a rectangular panel of material with one or two fastening straps on either side. This category includes the Knightrider harness, which can be secured around the wearer's lower abdomen or strapped onto a bed, chair, or other object. Because the Knightrider attaches at a single juncture and is equipped with long web straps, it is a good choice for really large individuals for whom neither a jockstrap-style nor a thong-style harness will fit.

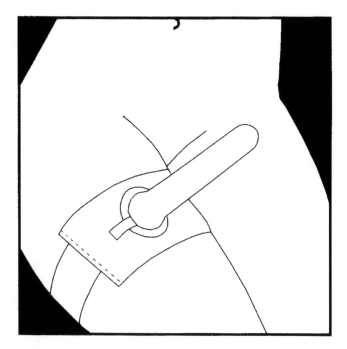

Illustration #6: Stormy Leather® Thigh One On Harness

Thigh harnesses are a standout in this category. These models are perfect for those times when you'd rather not evoke the notions of masculinity often associated with harnesses which situate a dildo on the wearer's pubic mound. These harnesses are made from leather, neoprene, or web material that forms a thick band around the wearer's thigh and holds a dildo against her leg. Many harness users enjoy this setup because the thigh is equipped with powerful muscles capable of both force and stamina. Thigh harnesses are also handy for seated positions—ambitious strappers can entertain two partners at the same time, with one riding each thigh. Another advantage to these models is that they leave the harness-wearer's vagina and anus completely unencumbered and accessible, enabling her to get her share of the action. Likewise, both partners can wear thigh harnesses to achieve simultaneous penetration. Thigh harnesses are also good for male strappers who want to try penetration from a new angle or who find it uncomfortable to strap a dildo over their genital area.

My all time favorite harness is Levi's 501 jeans. I think my butch looks way sexy in 'em. And I find that I experience the least amount of labial pinching from the 501s. Sure, sometimes those buttons can hit the wrong spot, but sometimes they hit the right spot.

The first time I had sex with a dildo and harness was in 1972. I was 17, sleeping with an older woman (she was 32). Sex toys were scarce in Humboldt, so we improvised with zucchini and duct tape.

Harness Material

Although leather is by far the material favored by most consumers, harnesses are also made from other materials such as nylon, webbing, neoprene, and even elastic, in the case of plastic dildos that come with straps attached. Leather has garnered its popularity because it molds to the body of the wearer over time, has an organic feel that many people enjoy, and is sturdy and visually appealing. Harnesses made from leather typically fasten with either D-rings or buckles. Though D-ring harnesses are quite adequate to the task, buckling harnesses are generally superior in strength and stability. D-ring harnesses work on a principle of tension; the straps are pulled through both rings, doubled back over one ring and under the other, and held in place by tightening the straps. This mechanism slightly damages the leather, though a well-made harness can withstand the stress. If a lot of slack remains after the harness has been fitted, the excess material can be cut off and the severed ends singed with a flame to prevent fraying. These harnesses range from $45 to $60.

If you're looking for a strong, durable harness that will hold a dildo snugly against your body and will last for a long time, you're on the right track with a leather buckling harness. Unlike leather D-ring harnesses, which are most often sewn together, buckling harnesses have rivets which hold the straps and buckles in place. The buckle preserves the integrity of the leather and provides for a nice fit. Buckles also allow you to don your harness quickly—simply store the harness with one side buckled and step in when you're ready for action. Buckling harnesses are generally made of thicker leather and are often augmented by decorative elements such as thick silver rings and functional features like an extra snap on the center strap to allow for a greater range of sizing options. The latter feature may be especially useful for shorter harness wearers who have difficulty with too much slack in the crotch area. These harnesses range from $70 to $100.

I strongly recommend spending a lot of money on a good harness. We use a Jewel Buckling harness from Stormy Leather, and it's great! The buckles are far superior to a D-ring harness (no slipping!).

What if you don't have a big wad of cash to plunk down for a fancy harness? Fear not—harnesses made

---

Dear Fairy Butch:

I'm a young dyke who just moved to San Francisco, and needless to say, I'm broke. Still, even us poor girls need to have our fun. I've got a dildo, but can you suggest a harness for those on a budget?

—Strapped on Sanchez

Dearest Strapped,

Well my dear, in no time at all you will be strapped in more ways than one. There is no reason those just starting out should be deprived of the pleasures a good harness can afford her. Neoprene/web harnesses are a great deal: they're cheap, sturdy, and washable! They are ideal for wearers just exploring dildo-harness sex, and are terrific "trick harnesses" for those gals with multiple partners. Expect to pay about 30 clams for one of these numbers, and you'll find it's money well spent.
XOXOXOXO,
Fairy Butch

from neoprene or webbing material are an excellent buy. These harnesses are cheap, sturdy, and washable. They are ideal for wearers who are just beginning to explore strap-on sex, vegans and others who prefer not to use animal products, and those with multiple partners who want to use a separate harness with each mate. Expect to spend between $30 to $40 for one of these models.

Try This on for Size

Ever been caught with your pants down—and no harness? If you are equipped with a lightweight dildo, such as a Cyberskin Realistic or moderately-sized PVC model, and some spare men's briefs, try this trick on for size. Start with three pairs of men's briefs. Your tighty whities should be good and snug—loosely fitting models just won't do. Make sure that they have a good thick, elastic waistband and a sturdy Y-front opening. Believe it or not, color makes a difference as well: bleached white undies tend to shrink down to a snug fit and maintain their tautness better than colored models, so they are your best bet. Once all three pairs are donned, put the bottom part of the flange or balls of the dildo directly up against your pubic mound, beneath the elastic waistband of the first pair of briefs. Then feed the tip of the dildo through the opening of the second pair of underwear, and finally through the third. If the toy is sufficiently lightweight and the undies acceptably snug, you should at this point have a dildo levitating out from your pelvis free of any visible means of support. This technique is also easily adapted to the purposes of packing. Just wear all three pairs of undies out the door and stick your toy against your skin, or between the first and second pairs for greater comfort. When that special moment arrives, just whip it out, feed it through, and you're ready for action!

Elastic is most often used in conjunction with a plastic dildo to form a prefabricated harness/dildo set or in a prosthetic penile appliance (PPA), a device designed to fit over a man's non-erect penis. These toys are useful for men who don't have an erection but want to involve their penis in the act of penetration. Unfortunately, most attached strap-on combination sets are mass-produced and of inferior quality, so be on the lookout for shoddy merchandise. The few exceptions are made of PVC or latex by reputable harness makers, such as Stormy Leather.

Dildo Harnessibility

So you've found a toy in a tantalizing shade of lipstick red, shaped like a lovely dolphin, and exactly the right size for your boyfriend's behind. Now you must pay attention to how the toy will work in a harness—it's time to determine its "harnessibility." To find a dildo that will best suit your needs, give heed to three factors: angle, flange, and firmness.

Angle of the Dangle

Determining the proper angle should be your first consideration. Dildos can be found in a wide range of angles, from skyscrapers to those that hang fully southward. Does the dildo you want have a sharp upward slope, a slight upward bend up, a fairly straight line, or a droop? Choose carefully, because along with the angle and height of your partner's body and that of your own, dildo curve is one of the five key variables involved in getting your toy to move where you want it to during strap-on sex. Since a sharp upward angle is prized among the naturally penised population, you might think that a similar geometry should be unfailingly emulated in their inanimate coun-

Dear Fairy Butch:

I am a novice at fucking women, and I have a hot date this coming weekend. I have a geometrical concern about the prospect. What is the proper angle, relative to the bed, I guess, at which to tilt a dildo for maximum G-spot satisfaction? I really want to make her happy.

—Would-be Studmuffin

Dear Woody,

And Darling, with a thoughtful and ambitious suitor such as yourself, happy is exactly what she shall be! Angle is indeed a crucial question in matters of the cunt, my dear, but you needn't dust off your 10th grade geometry book and protractor in order to bring pleasure to your amour.

Simply consider the position of the spot in question, *mon cherie.* The vaginal canal curves slightly up toward the cervix when she is on her back, and downwards when she is on hands and knees. It ensconces *le spot* about two to three inches inside the cooter on its front wall. Thus, when one is attempting to stimulate the little darling with your silicone (or rubber or polyurethane) peter, you should do your darndest to get it to emulate the curve of the lady at hand, or thereabouts.

You can do this in a variety of ways, Pet. For example, if you are approaching the damsel in the missionary position, then the desired curve would be upward. This can be achieved by either using a rigid silicone dildo with a more or less slightly upward curve, or by using a more floppy dildo in tandem with a snug jock strap and pair of boxers. If she's face down, simply lighten up on the support, angle the dildo down, and go about your business in a stunningly mathematically precise fashion.
XOXOXOXO,
Fairy Butch

terparts, but this is not so. Although a sharp upward tilt is terrific for some positions, there is no one perfect angle to search for when shopping for a dildo.

Consider which sexual positions interest you most. A dildo with a sharp skyward angle is well-suited for intense G-spot stimulation in the missionary position, while a toy that points downward works well for rear entry penetration. When either model is turned upside-down in a harness, however, it can be adapted to a variety of other positions—so if your budget allows for only one purchase, fret not. Similarly, a model that points straight out can be adaptable to a variety of positions—just use the elastic band of your undergarment to manipulate the dildo's angle. (See Chapter 8, Packing)

Flange Facts

The base of the dildo from which the shaft originates is called the flange; this is the part that holds the toy in place in a harness. It is crucial that the dildo flange be large enough to ensure that the toy does not come through the O-ring of the harness during use. You can test the effectiveness of the flange by placing the dildo in the harness and giving it a good tug to make sure that it does not come through the O-ring.

If the flange of the toy is not wide enough for your harness, you have two choices. If your harness comes with a removable O-ring, you can substitute a smaller O-ring. Or you can purchase a SlipNot adapter to extend the size of the flange. The adapter enlarges the diameter of the flange and holds the dildo steady in the harness, making the movements of the toy more consistent with your own. Other flange features to consider are comfort—how does it feel pressed into your pubic mound?—and its potential for providing you with stimulation. Some flanges have a rippled surface on the side facing the wearer to provide her with clitoral stimulation during strap-on sex.

The Firmness Factor

One final factor in evaluating the harnessibility of a toy is its firmness. While some people prefer soft toys, particularly for anal use, properly-sized firm toys often provide less friction against the vaginal or anal walls. In addition, firm toys move more readily with the body of the harness wearer, whereas soft toys tend to have a mind of their own. On the other hand, softer dildos are especially comfortable for packing (wearing a dildo underneath your clothing).

Care and Feeding: Lubricant, Latex, and Toy Cleaning

5

"Safety First" was likely the motto espoused by your high school driving instructor, and caution and courtesy are similarly consequential in strap-on sex. Lubricant, latex, and lather will help pave the road to strap-on success. Keeping your toys clean and covering them in latex will help prevent the spread of sexually-transmitted diseases (STDs) and lessen the occurrence of infections of all sorts. Proper care will increase the life of your toys, as well as the likelihood of a second date. Lubricant can make a not-so-good thing great and a great thing last longer.

Condom Consciousness

We've all heard the maxim "an ounce of prevention is worth a pound of cure," and in the context of strap-on sex, that translates to using latex barriers. Latex condoms can remedy some of the ills associated with the use of Cyberskin, PVC, soft plastic, latex, and mystery rubber toys by preventing the abrasion of these materials with friction. This reduces the transmission of microorganisms between partners. Unlike silicone, these materials cannot be disinfected in boiling water and can trap germs in their larger pores.

Even when using silicone toys, there are plenty of good reasons to keep condoms on hand. Just because silicone can be disinfected doesn't mean this option will always be convenient for you. Say you've donned your dildo and done your partner six ways to Sunday and now want her to penetrate you. With an uncovered dildo, you would have to disinfect it prior to making the switch. With condoms, all you have to do is strip one off and put a fresh one on, and you're ready for the about-face.

Or perhaps you are tempted to go a knocking at your date's backdoor after you've been well received at the front. If you later wish to resume vaginal penetration, you can quickly put on a new condom rather than disinfecting the toy you just used in her ass. Remember: anal flora must never be introduced into the vagina, even when the anus and vagina belong to the same person. (Anal bacteria can cause vaginal infections.) Finally, condoms are beneficial if you will be having an extended bout of strap-on sex with breaks between rounds of penetration. After you take the toy out of your partner, dust particles will stick to its moist surface and it will not be fit for further use. A quick condom switch will help you practice both safer sex and good hygiene.

Pay attention to the material of the condoms you purchase. Latex condoms are most widely available. Polyurethane condoms are a good choice for those who are sensitive to latex. However, condoms made from animal products, like lambskin, are not; STDs can pass through the larger pores of condoms made from animal membranes. Also note whether the condom has a pre-applied lubricant. Some people are sensitive to nonoxynol-9 and similar products found in lubricated condoms; you may prefer to purchase unlubricated condoms and use a lubricant of your own choosing.

Glove Your Love

Exploration by hand is an essential prelude to good strap-on sex. Just as you wrap condoms on your toys, you should consider the use of gloves on your hands. Latex gloves can help protect you and your partner in a variety of ways. First, latex gloves help prevent the transmission of certain STDs by creating a barrier between the semen, vaginal fluids, or blood of one partner and any fissures such as hangnails or paper cuts on the hands of the other. For example, gloves can help reduce the spread of herpes and genital warts—a person who has had contact with a partner's genitals or anus can remove the glove prior to touching her own genitals, anus, mouth, or other mucous membranes. Finally, gloves can help prevent vaginal infection by interrupting the transit of anal bacteria to the vagina. Simply peel off the glove used for anal penetration and replace it with a fresh one before touching the vulva. Resourceful individuals may wear one glove on top of the other so they can travel from anus to vagina—or from partner to partner—in seconds.

If the virtues of gloves were limited to their role in better hygiene and safer sex, this would be sufficient incentive to buy them in volume. But gloves also improve the aerodynamics of manual penetration. Gloves keep things slippery longer because they prevent lubricant from being absorbed into the wearer's skin. They also cover any drag-producing hangnails or patches of rough skin. Likewise, those with long nails can wear gloves with cotton balls in the fingertips. For best results, choose an appropriately sized glove and put a bit of lubricant inside to heighten your own sensitivity as you stroke your partner. You can stock up on generic latex gloves at drug stores and warehouse clubs. If you are sensitive to latex, try the hypo allergenic non-latex variety found at medical supply houses or sex stores.

Keeping It Clean

Dildos

Silicone: Clean silicone toys with warm water, a mild antibacterial soap or toy cleaner such as Hibiclens or ForPlay Adult Toy Cleanser, and a gentle food scrubber. Silicone dildos can be disinfected by washing them in bleach rinse, placing them in the top rack of a dishwasher, or boiling them in water for up to five minutes. If your silicone dildo has a built-in vibrator, remove the vibrating portion before disinfecting. Wash the vibrator separately with warm water and an antibacterial soap, making sure to keep the battery pack dry. To prevent corrosion, vibrating eggs can be placed in a finger cot before inserting them into the dildo. For longer battery and vibrator life, store batteries outside the toy. Store silicone toys in a toy sack or thick sock, and keep them away from sharp edges. When traveling, protect silicone toys from the edges of toiletry bottles and other sharp items in your luggage. Never use silicone-based lubricants with silicone toys.

Cyberskin: Because Cyberskin readily attracts dirt and dust, condoms are highly recommended. Be especially meticulous with storage, and keep them away from ink

A Tip from Fairy Butch

There's little I love more than a relaxing bath. I could spend hours in the warm water, soaking up the aromatherapy bath oil and applying my three-part facial. Oh, how I rue the day I signed a lease for *un petit chateau sans* bathtub. Alas. Though I realize there is little hope for me in my tragic state of affairs, my sex toys do not suffer the same fate. And though I am happy to care for them properly, it is difficult to suppress the occasional *soupçon* of longing as I guide them through the following bathing ritual:

1. Procure a gargantuan soup pot, fill it with water, and bring to a boil.
2. Submerge several silicone toys in the boiling water and let them boil for about three minutes. Use a wooden utensil or wooden tongs to retrieve them, and be careful not to hold them up against the hot surface of the metal when fishing them out of the mix. (You can re-use the same water for all your silicone toys.)
3. Run them under cold water until they are cool enough to touch. You can hold them under the faucet with tongs or toss them into a sieve. Set the toys on a clean towel to air dry or pat dry.
4. Stash your clean toys in a toy bag or cloth-lined drawer to prevent them from attracting dirt and dust.
5. Repeat the process until all your silicone toys have been cleaned.
6. Allow the water to cool until it is hot but not boiling. You can add some cold water if you are in a rush. Add the appropriate amount of ForPlay Adult Toy Cleanser (the bottle is labeled with a handy measuring grid) and swirl the mix around with your utensil (no, darling, I mean the wooden spatula.) Don't be too concerned about the nonoxynol-9 in the cleaner unless you are super-sensitive—you'll be rinsing it off later, cupcake.

7. Now drop your non-silicone toys into the water. If there is room at the top of the pot, position your battery-operated vibrators so that the business end of the toy is submerged but the battery pack is nowhere near the water.

8. Soak the non-silicone toys in the hot water for about 20 minutes.

9. Take a gentle bristle food scrubber and lightly scrub the surface of the soaking darlings.

10. Rinse well and set to dry on a clean towel.

11. When the pot is devoid of toys, use the hot water to scrub the contact surfaces of your electric vibes with the food scrubber, daintily avoiding the remainder of the toy in a lady-like fashion.

12. Harnesses may be cleaned with the food scrubber dipped in the warm water mixture. Take care not to use too much of the water and cleaner. Air dry.

And there you have it, Sweet Cheeks, just the thing to perk up those little lolly-gagging lovelies lying about your *pied-à-terre*.

and dyed clothing. Clean Cyberskin toys with warm water and a mild antibacterial cleaner such as Hibiclens or ForPlay Adult Toy Cleanser. Lather the soap in your hands, work over the toy, rinse, and pat dry with a cloth towel. Cyberskin dildos cannot be disinfected. Before storing these toys, dust them with cornstarch and place in a toy sack or a thick sock. Rinse off the cornstarch prior to use. Do not dust with talcum powder.

Latex: Clean latex toys with warm water, a mild antibacterial cleaner like Hibiclens or ForPlay Adult Toy Cleanser, and a gentle food scrubber. These items cannot be disinfected. Store in a cool, dry place, and do not expose to sunlight. Latex may break down after extended use. Never use any type of oil-based product with latex toys.

Mystery rubber, PVC, and soft plastic: Clean dildos made from these materials with warm water, a mild antibacterial cleaner such as Hibiclens or ForPlay Adult Toy Cleanser, and a gentle food scrubber. If your dildo is equipped with a vibrator, remove the vibrating portion before cleaning if possible, and be sure to keep the battery unit dry. Dildos made of these materials cannot be disinfected, and condoms are highly recommended. Store your toys in a toy sack or a thick sock, and keep them away from ink and dyed clothing.

Harnesses

Leather: Clean leather harnesses with warm water, a mild antibacterial soap or toy cleaner, and a washcloth; do not submerge them in water. Use leather cleanser for an occasional buffing. Leather harnesses cannot be disinfected; the highest level of cleansing can be achieved with adult toy cleaners containing nonoxynol-9. Allow harnesses to air dry away from direct sunlight. After harnesses have dried completely, store in a cool, dark place.

Neoprene: These harnesses do not conform to the wearer's body as leather does, but they are an excellent choice for users who want a harness that can be readily disinfected. Clean neoprene harnesses with warm water, a mild antibacterial soap or toy cleaner, and a washcloth. They can also be machine-washed on the gentle cycle. Allow harnesses to air dry completely, and store them in a cool, dark place.

Smooth Sailing

Lubricant, like money, isn't worth much on its own, but a little lube sure does make the best things in life go more smoothly. In fact, most sex acts can be improved with a bit of the wet stuff: lubricants can prolong strap-on sex and help transform painful intercourse into pleasure.

Water-based lubricants have been selling at record rates in recent years, with each lubricant company introducing new variations on the theme each sales season. Yet some people are reluctant to use lubricants. Some women and their partners regard copious vaginal lubrication as a sign of sexual arousal in women, much as an unflagging hard-on is in men. They believe that if a woman is *truly* aroused, she will produce sufficient vaginal lubrication for comfortable penetration. In fact, many variables affect the amount and consistency of vaginal fluid a woman will produce, including age, diet, use of alcohol or drugs, and stage of the menstrual cycle. Commercial lubricants are beneficial when a woman's natural secretions are too sparse or too thick to achieve a good pace for thrusting without uncomfortable friction, and can be especially useful during extended strap-on sex after natural lubrication has been depleted. As for anal sex, since the anus produces very little natural lubrication, additional lubricant is a must to protect the delicate mucous membranes that line the rectum.

Which kind of lubricant is best suited for strap-on sex? While some sexual.virtuosos favor oils, creams, and lotions to reduce the friction of sexual activity, these substances generally leave much to be desired compared to water-based lubricants. Oils are difficult to remove from the vagina (and can lead to vaginal infections), tend to attract dirt and germs, and are incompatible with latex barriers and toys. Scented products designed for external

Dear Fairy Butch:
   I'm not sure how I feel about using artificial lubricant.
Shouldn't I be able to get wet enough on my own?
                                        —Golden Gate Granola Girl

Dear Fairy Butch:
   Would you please pontificate on the pleasures of lube?
                                        —Slippery in Santa Fe

Darlings,

   Some gals feel that if they can't produce sufficient
vaginal fluids to enable their favorite sexual activities, then
they are in some way inadequate to the task—they aren't
turned on enough, or aren't "woman" enough to partake in
the fun. I say, *au contraire,* my Pet! Though arousal is indeed
a function of lubrication, there are many elements which
can influence the process as well: age, menstrual cycle, and
diet, to name a few. These factors can also effect the
consistency of the mix as well, making the fluid too thick to
get up a good pace without uncomfortable friction. In
addition, some folks like to go to the well more than one
time in a sitting, and use up the bodily-produced stuff in
the first round.

   Whatever the situation, there are few occasions which
couldn't benefit from a *soupçon* of the wet stuff. Get thee to
a pharmacy!
XOXOXOX,
Fairy Butch

use can irritate the delicate membranes of the anus and vagina, and lotions and creams may be absorbed too quickly into the skin to prevent abrasion during intercourse. While water-based lubricants do tend to dry out with friction and exposure to the air, they can be revived by adding a bit of saliva or warm water. Some fans of water-based lube keep a spray bottle on hand for this purpose.

Fairy Butch's Guide to Lube Selection

There are many brands of water-based lubricants available, and the sheer number throws many strap-on sex customers into a quandary. You can expedite the selection process by considering the following:

1. your preferences in taste and texture,
2. any skin sensitivities or allergies you or your partner may have,
3. the specific demands of the sexual activity you have in mind.

Many people with sensitive skin do well with water-based lubricants, but have problems with nonoxynol-9, a spermicide used in many varieties. Some lube users find that nonoxynol-9 leads to skin irritations. Other folks have trouble with products that contain glycerin, which may encourage yeast infections.

The process of matching a lubricant to a particular sex act is somewhat subjective. Lubricants can be classified in terms of thickness vs. thinness and cohesiveness vs. viscosity. We all think of lubes in terms of thickness and thinness; to think in terms of cohesiveness (facilitating movement) and viscosity (staying put) is a new concept for most people. Cohesive lubes have a consistency that is especially good for promoting rapid movement during penetration, while viscous lubes cling to the walls of the vagina or rectum. If you are fisting your partner's vagina or penetrating her ass with a dildo, for instance, you will likely want to use a lube that will coat the walls of the orifice *and stay there.* You'll want a viscous lube. If the action speeds up, you can add a more slippery lube to the mix. Cohesive lubes promote movement.

Super-slick emollient lubricants like Astroglide, Probe, Liquid Silk, and ID are great for gaining speed in vaginal thrusting. For anal sex, however, you may want to start off by coating the anus and rectum with a heavy, viscous lube like Maximus, Embrace, or ForPlay, then add a slicker lube as things heat up.

Silicone lubricants are long-lasting and feel oily (although they are *not* oil-based). They are tasteless, transfer heat, do not dry out, and do not contain glycerin. However, they are highly flammable, leave greasy stains, cannot be used safely with silicone toys, and are not well-tolerated by some people with certain skin sensitivities. Silicone lubricants are also very expensive. They will, however, combine nicely with water-based lube. You can get more bang for your buck (and the best of both worlds) by creating your own mixture of the two. Add a teaspoon of silicone lube to a 5-ounce bottle of water-based lube. Shake vigorously before each use.

Here is a handy guide to choosing lube for strap-on sex, complete with ratings for viscosity to cohesiveness (on a 1 to 10 scale, 1 is most cohesive and 10 is most viscous) and thinness to thickness (on a 1 to 10 scale, 1 is thinnest and 10 is thickest).

AquaLube: Slightly waxy, becomes tacky as it dries and does not last long with friction. Pleasant coconut flavor. Contains many ingredients, which can increase the risk of chemical sensitivities. Cohesiveness/Viscosity: 4. Thinness/Thickness: 2.

Astroglide: Very thin, slick, light, adherent; tends to dry out with friction and exposure to air, but can be easily revived with water or saliva. Has a slightly sweet taste because it contains glycerin. Sports a glow-in-the dark label. Cohesiveness/Viscosity: 2. Thinness/Thickness: 2.

Born Again: Separates easily; highly viscous and very tacky. Chemical taste similar to rubber cement. Contains wild yam extract and vitamin E; marketed to post-menopausal women as a moisturizing gel. Light brown color. Cohesiveness/Viscosity: 7. Thinness/Thickness: 7.

Embrace Regular: Very thick, non-adherent, separates easily, becomes tacky as it dries, and clings well to vaginal and anal walls. Has a slightly sweet taste. Good for anal sex and fisting. Contains saccharin and artificial dyes. Cohesiveness/Viscosity: 8. Thinness/Thickness: 10.

Embrace Strawberry: Very thick, non-adherent; separates easily; becomes tacky as it dries; clings well to vaginal and anal walls. Has a slightly sweet, light, strawberry flavor. Good for anal sex and fisting. Contains saccharin and artificial dyes. Cohesiveness/Viscosity: 8. Thinness/Thickness: 10.

Eros: Extremely thin, tasteless, does not dry, transfers heat readily. This lube is silicone-based and should not be used with silicone toys. It's flammable and prone to stains, so spills should be cleaned immediately with soap and water. Not well-tolerated by some people with certain skin sensitivities. Cohesiveness/Viscosity: 7. Thinness/Thickness: 1.

ForPlay Personal Lubricant: Very thick and viscous; has a waxy feel when wet, leaves a bit of residue when dry; stays fairly wet over time. Tastes like powdered sugar. Good for anal sex and fisting because it clings well to vaginal and anal walls. Cohesiveness/Viscosity: 7. Thinness/Thickness: 7.

ForPlay with nonoxynol-9: Very thick and viscous; has a waxy feel when wet, leaves a bit of residue when dry; stays somewhat wet over time. Has an acrid taste. Contains nonoxynol-9; should be wiped off with a warm cloth prior to oral sex because of the unpleasant taste and the tongue-numbing effect of the spermicide. Cohesiveness/Viscosity: 7. Thinness/Thickness: 7.

ForPlay Succulents: Has a waxy feel; gets warm when blown on. Five favors, mostly fruits. The Passion Fruit has slight aftertaste; the Peach has a pleasant taste. Contains a large amount of glycerin. Folks who may not have problems with the lessor amounts of glycerin in other lubes may nonetheless have problems with this product. Marketed especially for oral sex. Cohesiveness/Viscosity: 7. Thinness /Thickness: 6.

ID Glide: Stays very slick with exposure to air, cohesive but not stringy, ideal for vaginal strap-on sex. Has a slightly sweet taste due to the fact that it contains glycerin. Cohesiveness/Viscosity: 3. Thinness/Thickness: 5.

ID Juicy Lubes: Stays very wet. Several flavors: cherry, peach, and watermelon get a higher rating for taste appeal than mint and piña colada. Contains glycerin, saccharin, and aspartame; not recommended for women who are prone to vaginal infections. Avoid contact with ears and eyes. Cohesiveness/Viscosity: 2. Thinness/Thickness: 7.

ID Millennium: Extremely thin, tasteless, does not dry, transfers heat readily. This lube is silicone-based and should not be used with silicone toys. It's flammable and prone to stains, so spills should be cleaned immediately with soap and water. Not well-tolerated by some people with certain skin sensitivities. Cohesiveness/Viscosity: 7. Thinness/Thickness: 1.

Just Between Us: Very stringy and waxy, stays wet and slippery, tasteless, and leaves a slight residue. This product is 50 percent aloe vera and contains glycerin. CohesivenessViscosity: 7. ThinnessThickness: 7.

KY Liquid: Becomes thicker with exposure to air, leaves a residue as it dries. Slightly sweet, with an aftertaste. Glycerin is the first ingredient listed on the label; check the expiration date on the container. Cohesiveness/Viscosity: 2. Thinness/Thickness: 1.

Liquid Silk: Non-drying, non-tacky, and opaque; stays extremely wet and slippery. Has a bitter, medicinal taste. You might want to wipe off with a warm cloth prior to oral sex because of the unpleasant taste. Does not contain glycerin. Cohesiveness/Viscosity: 2. Thinness/Thickness: 5.

Maximus: Thick, waxy and non-drying; maintains its slipperiness as it clings well to vaginal and anal walls. Has a bitter, medicinal taste. You might want to wipe off with a warm cloth prior to oral sex because of the unpleasant taste. Great for anal sex and fisting. Does not contain glycerin. Cohesiveness/Viscosity: 4. Thinness/Thickness: 8.

Pour Venus: Extremely thin, tasteless, does not dry, transfers heat readily. This lube is silicone-based and should not be used with silicone toys. It's flammable and prone to stains, so spills should be cleaned immediately with soap and water. Not well-tolerated by some people with certain skin sensitivities. Cohesiveness/Viscosity: 7. Thinness/Thickness: 1.

Probe Silky Light: Stays wet after exposure to air, becomes stringy with friction. This tasteless lube is one of the most natural lubricants on the market. It's good for people with chemical sensitivities, although it does contains vegetable glycerin; also contains grapefruit seed extract which can be spermicidal. Don't use if you want to get pregnant. Cohesiveness/Viscosity: 4. Thinness/Thickness: 3.

Probe Thick Rich: Stays wet after exposure to air, becomes stringy with friction. This tasteless lube is one of the most natural lubricants on the market. It's good for people with chemical sensitivities, although it does contains vegetable glycerin; also contains grapefruit seed extract which can be spermicidal. Don't use if you want to get pregnant. Cohesiveness/Viscosity: 3. Thinness/Thickness: 6.

Slippery Stuff Gel: Stays wet with use, but gets tacky as it dries. Tasteless. Does not contain glycerin. Cohesiveness/Viscosity: 7. Thinness/Thickness: 7.

Slippery Stuff Liquid: Extremely liquid; pours out rapidly. Tasteless. Does not contain glycerin. Cohesiveness/Viscosity: 2. Thinness/Thickness: 1.

Dear Fairy Butch,
Any hints on keeping my lube handy? The bottle seems to
roll off the bed at just the wrong moment!
—Dried Up in Dallas

Dear Dried Up,
Have you ever been elbow deep in some lovely creature while she's moaning and screaming out the lyrics to La Traviata as you pump steadily inside her? Has your latex glove ever started to feel as dry as the Sahara? Have you grappled furiously for the lube, only to discover that your Astroglide is nowhere to be found?
Try this handy dandy tip next time, Sugar. Put some Velcro on each of two lube bottles, and a bit more on each bedpost or on each side of the bed frame. Slap the bottles on the bed, put your girlie between the sheets, and luxuriate in the knowledge that you're primed and ready to go.
No more lost lube bottle for you!
XOXOXOXO,
Fairy Butch

Down and Dirty: Positions for Strap-on Sex

Now that we have explored anatomy, dildos, harnesses, and sex-toy cleaning, it's time to saddle up and take aim. This chapter discusses strap-on sex positions. Although the mechanics involved in each position generally work similarly for both anal and vaginal penetration, some exceptions are noted. While this chapter includes enough sexual formations to keep you busy for a month of Sundays, it's only a jumping off point. Feel free to improvise. So pick a position, get the basics, note the precautions, experiment with the variations, and happy pumping!

The Missionary Position

The missionary position, a time-honored standby, is actually an umbrella term for a variety of postures, all of which situate the receptive partner on his or her back with the insertive partner on top. This position allows for face-to-face contact and a great deal of pelvic stimulation for both partners.

Eye to eye. Face to face. Tit to tit. Belly to belly. Bush to bush. Push.

In the standard version of the missionary position, the insertive partner is on top and facing the receptive partner. The insertive partner is positioned between her partner's spread legs, and the receptive partner's legs are straight with his heels on the surface of the bed. Alternatively, the receptive partner can bend her knees and place her feet flat on the bed, which allows her to better control her hips and meet the thrusts of her partner. Likewise, the receptive partner can raise her hips higher than her head by placing a pillow or two beneath her hips.

The walls of the receptive partner's vagina and anus are compressed when she raises her legs at a higher angle. This creates a tighter squeeze around the dildo, providing more friction and more intense G-spot or prostate stimulation. For even more direct stimulation, the receptive partner can prop his or her legs up on the insertive partner's shoulders. This variation endows the insertive partner with a high degree of responsibility because she has control of both the angle and the depth of her thrusts. Strappers who try this variation should be fairly experienced and able to read their partner's responses. This alternative requires more strength on the part of the strapper, and can place a high degree of strain on the receptive partner's lower back. Placing just one leg on the insertive partner's shoulder and leaving the other leg bent with the foot flat on the bed can provide the receptive partner with more control and less lower back strain. The missionary position can be adapted for anal sex by raising the hips even more.

Dear Fairy Butch,

I love fucking my girlfriend with my dildo and harness in the missionary position, but with her legs spread wide and up in the air, so that I can really hit her G-spot when I thrust into her. The only thing is that though she enjoys this way of doing things as much as I do, it's hard for her to hold her legs up for very long. Any ideas?

—Curious in Cleveland

Darling Curious,

I feel your pain (not to mention that of your girlfriend). I have just the ticket for you: ankle restraints. But this time, try them in this newfangled trick I came up with to suit just this purpose. In this advanced position, the receptive partner wears ankle restraints, the rings of which are tethered to the bedpost or futon frame behind her head. This allows you to position her legs at an angle which is particularly conducive to intense G-spot stimulation, and relieves her from the often tiresome necessity of either holding her own legs up in the air or having you hold them up for her. Needless to say, this posture requires some masterful dildo and harness handling on your part.

Allow me to throw a few provisos your way though before you trot on down to ye local leather tannery. First of all, folks with lower back injuries may find this position painful. Likewise, the receptive partner is quite vulnerable in this position, and it should be undertaken only in an atmosphere of trust. If the prospect of having both legs immobilized feels painful to your girlfriend, or overwhelming for either of you, experiment with tying up only one leg, or propping up her legs by placing pillows at her sides underneath them. In any case, happy strappin', Papi!

XOXOXOXO,

Fairy Butch

Fucking a boy with my dick is one of my favorite things to do. I like to lay him on his back so I can look into his eyes while the base of my dildo presses into my clit.

My ass is against the windshield of a VW Bug, and her legs are over my shoulders, with her feet against the windshield.

In the thigh harness adaptation of the missionary position, the receptive partner lies on her back with her legs spread. The strapper leans over her with her harnessed thigh between her partner's legs, while she balances her weight on her palms and the non-harnessed thigh.

The Rear-Entry Position

Due to its essential appeal, as well as its frequent appearance in erotic literature and films, the rear-entry position is a popular feature in the sex lives of many strap-on devotees. Like the missionary position, the rear-entry or "doggy style" posture is an umbrella term for a variety of positions, all of which situate both partners facing the same direction with the receptive partner face down and the insertive partner behind and/or on top of the receptive partner. This position gives the strapper a great deal of access to his or her partner's body and allows for deep vaginal or anal penetration.

The standard rear-entry position has the receptive partner on all fours with the insertive partner behind him, holding onto his hips for leverage. To assist the insertive partner in controlling the angle of the dildo, the receptive partner should keep her head lower than her hips and arch her back so that her anus or vagina is angled upward toward her partner.

My favorite position is from behind because I like the slapping sound.

There are several possible variations on the rear-entry position. Rather than kneeling on the bed behind her partner, the strapper can place one foot on the bed and leave her other knee down. This facilitates deeper penetration and offers a greater degree of leverage and thrusting power for many people. Another variation begins much like the standard stance. After the insertive partner enters his or her partner from behind, she can move on top in a parallel position and lay directly atop the receptive partner's body. This variation allows for a full-body embrace and offers both partners a firm surface against which to grind, which can provide a great deal of clitoral or penile stimulation. The insertive partner can wrap her legs tightly around the legs of her partner to gain even greater friction and genital stimulation.

To intensify the power dynamics that are often associated with the rear-entry position, the strapper can grasp the forearms or wrists of his partner and pull him or her back onto his dildo while thrusting. This variation helps situate the receptive partner at a favorable angle for G-spot or prostate stimulation. It requires a great deal of trust between partners because the strapper has more control over the activity, yet is unable to see the expression on his partner's face. People with repetitive stress injuries or otherwise weak wrists or arms should avoid this variation.

The Side-by-Side Position

The side-by-side position is a wonderful setup for receptive partners who are pregnant or for partners of dissimilar size. The standard side-by-side position places both partners in a spoon position with the strapper behind his or her partner. The receptive partner can arch her back to help ease the dildo into her vagina or anus while the insertive partner holds onto her hips and thrusts. Although this position is not ideal for vigorous thrusting, each partner's body is fully supported by the bed, and it allows for a great deal of body-to-body contact, letting the partners kiss, snuggle, or stimulate each other's torsos or genitals during strap-on sex. The strapper can extend her endurance by alternating between thrusting and rocking the insertive partner back and forth on the dildo.

> The doggy-style and missionary positions always require more care than the side-by-side style. I like the scissors position best because I can concentrate on enjoyment when there is nothing stopping my strokes.

There are many possible variations to the side-by-side position. For example, the receptive partner can gain leverage by facing her mate, draping a leg over the legs of her partner, placing her foot flat on the surface behind him, and thrusting onto the dildo. Another tech-

Common Sense for Shorter Strappers

Here's a terrific adaptation for insertive partners who are much shorter than their mates. You and your partner lie side by side, facing one another. Place her thigh over your shoulder. You can reach her vagina or anus with your hand for a warm-up, and then penetrate her vaginally or anally with your strap-on. With her thigh raised, her anus and vagina are compressed, providing an advantageous angle for G-spot (or prostrate) stimulation. Because her thigh is raised over your shoulder, the difference in your heights is equalized.

nique lets thigh harness users enjoy simultaneous penetration. The partners face one another and straddle each others' harness-equipped thighs. They can embrace while using the strength of their legs to thrust into one another. This position allows both partners to enjoy clitoral or penile stimulation by rubbing their genitals on their partner's thigh. In an anal adaptation of the side-by-side position, the receptive partner brings her legs up to her chest while her partner spoons her and enters her from behind. The insertive partner can gain greater leverage in this posture by placing one foot on the surface of the bed.

The Receptive Partner on Top Position

Positions that place the receptive partner on top offer her a great deal of control over the depth and angle of thrusts into her vagina or anus. Additionally, the insertive partner can provide direct clitoral, penile, or anal stimulation with his hands and can stroke his partner's breasts, ass, or back, depending on whether the receptive partner is facing or turned away from him. Because of the increased mobility, partners can easily thrust in rhythm with one another. If the partners face one another, there is added visual stimulation. Because it is easier for the receptive partner to slide all the way down onto the dildo rather than cut her thrusting short, it is particularly important in this position to choose a dildo of appropriate length. The insertive partner will have more control over her thrusts if she bends her knees and places her feet flat on the surface of the bed rather than lying with her legs extended. In the standard receptive partner on top position, the insertive partner lies on her back with her legs bent and her feet flat on the bed. The receptive partner straddles his or her mate and mounts the dildo.

In a variation of this position, the receptive partner turns away from her mate and faces her feet. The strapper grasps her partner's hips and helps her move in rhythm to her thrusts. Though the strapper can enjoy watching from this vantage point, the receptive partner's vision is limited. Make sure that the angle of the dildo is adjusted to accommodate changes in the curve of the receptive partner's vagina or anus as she turns around.

In another variation, the receptive partner squats onto the dildo rather than kneeling astride her partner. This position enables the receptive partner to use the entire muscular structure of her legs to thrust onto the dildo. The strapper can help her maintain her balance by holding her partner in place. To make her anus more accessible in this position, the receptive partner can lean back with her palms behind her and thrust her hips upward. The squatting position shifts a lot of weight onto the receptive partner's knees, and is therefore inadvisable for people with joint problems.

In the thigh harness adaptation of this position, the strapper lies on the bed with a thigh harness strapped in place and his partner mounts his harnessed thigh, facing in either direction. Again, be sure to adjust the angle of the dildo to correspond with the curve of the receptive partner's anus or vagina.

When I use a dildo, I like to lie on my back and have my husband sit on it; it's easier for me to control that way.

The Sitting Position

In the sitting position, the strapper is seated with the receptive partner straddling his or her legs with the dildo inside her vagina or anus. The partners can easily thrust in rhythm with one another and enjoy ample body contact. This position is easily adaptable to excitingly furtive situations such as car sex or antics in a suburban mall men's room. In the sitting position, it is especially important to choose a dildo of the appropriate length, because it is easier for the receptive partner to slide fully down onto the dildo than to moderate his or her movements up and down.

The standard version of this position situates the receptive partner facing the strapper and straddling his lap, kneeling on the surface upon which he is seated. The insertive partner sits with his legs together and the dildo propped up between them while the receptive partner mounts the toy. The insertive partner will have more control and power in his thrusting if he bends his knees and places his feet flat on the surface, rather than extending his legs in front of him.

As an alternative, the receptive partner may turn and face the other direction rather than facing her mate. The strapper can help the receptive partner lift her hips and move her body in rhythm with the insertive partner's thrusts. Be certain though to adjust the angle of the dildo to accommodate changes in the curve of the receptive partner's vagina or anus as she turns around. Though the strapper has a full view of the dildo moving in and out of her mate, the receptive partner's vision is limited in this position.

In another variation, the receptive partner stands on the surface upon which her mate is seated and squats onto the dildo, facing either forward or backward. In this position the receptive partner can use the strength of her legs to thrust onto the dildo, and the strapper can hold onto her partner's hips to help her maintain her balance. This position puts a great deal of stress on the receptive partner's knees, making it inadvisable for those with joint problems.

In a thigh harness variation of the sitting position, the strapper sits with a thigh harness strapped into place. The receptive partner either kneels and straddles her mate's thighs, or squats down onto the dildo for greater leverage. She may face either direction, as long as the angle of the dildo is adjusted to conform with the curve of her anus or vagina.

The Standing Position

In the standing position, both partners stand facing each other or facing in the same direction, usually with one leaning against a wall for added balance and leverage. Although this position is acrobatic and taxing, it is favored by many for the sense of urgency it lends to strap-on sex, evoking the fervency of a back-alley quickie.

The standard version of this position has the receptive partner leaning with her back against a wall. Her legs are spread wide enough to allow the insertive partner to enter her, but not so wide that her vulva and anus are too low for her partner to access them. The strapper enters his mate and wraps his hands around her hips. Either partner can bring his or her legs closer together or further apart to adjust for differences in height. The standing position works best if both partners, but particularly the strapper, develop lower-body strength. Building up your quadriceps (front thighs), hamstrings (back thighs), and gluteus maximus (butt) muscles can help you gain agility and endurance for this position. Most forms of aerobic activity improve leg strength, but for more a more dramatic increase in strength, try resistance exercises such as leg presses or squats.

My favorite position is from the back, my fag dyke boy grasping a fence.

There are many variations on the standing position. One option has the receptive partner turn around to face the wall. Make certain to adjust the angle of the dildo as he changes direction. In this alternative, the strapper has greater freedom to grab her partner's hips and thrust into her. To make this position amenable to anal sex, the receptive partner can stabilize himself against the wall and arch his back. Using a chair can make this position easier to achieve for both partners, since the receptive partner can support his body weight by leaning over the chair and holding onto its back. This helps him readily arch his back and spread his legs to find a comfortable fit for penetration.

In a more advanced version of the standing position, the strapper faces his mate and holds her against the wall. The receptive partner spreads her legs and hooks them around the strapper's upper arms or back. She can stabilizes herself by wrapping her arms tightly around her mate's neck and pushing back against the wall. The strapper must stand far enough away from the wall to lower his partner into a position that allows for penetration. This variation requires a great deal of strength on the part of the strapper and considerable flexibility on the part of the receptive partner. Likewise, the strapper must take care to prevent banging her partner's head against the wall.

I love to strap a dildo to my lover's back so I can go for a "horsie ride." Crop and spurs not necessary.

Keep Your Mojo Working: Geometry, Timing & Staying Power

The experience of novice strappers pounding their toys into the perineum of their partners, or of giving them too much G-spot or prostate stimulation too soon, has left many a dildo-and-harness rig gathering dust in their owner's toy box. To avoid such calamity, it is vital that every strapper have some knowledge of anatomy. This includes generic anatomical comprehension as well as idiosyncrasies particular to each partner's body and preferences in type and rate of stimulation during strap-on sex, along with the mechanics involved in bringing these effects to fruition. Specific anatomical inquiries can be directed to Chapter 2, Anatomy: Learning the Lay of the Land, and communication pointers are detailed in Chapter 13, Bringing It Home: Communicating with Your Partner. But where can you go to develop a knowledge of the mechanics of strap-on sex, as well as methods of developing the stamina to do the deed? Give heed to the following tips on strap-on geometry and other allied topics to fill the gap. Though its title may have you reaching for compass and protractor, rest assured that the results of your study will be more fruitful than in 10th-grade math class.

Stamina

Increasing your strength and aerobic capacity will enable you to better enjoy strap-on sex, regardless of which side of the dildo you find yourself on. It may seem strange to exercise in order to gain more satisfaction from sex, but I can't think of better motivation to take a turn on the treadmill.

Physical exercise of all kinds can enhance your sexual experiences. Developing a greater aerobic capacity will help you feel less exhausted during a rousing bout of in-and-out, and you will find that you can enjoy sex for a longer period of time. Stretching promotes greater flexibility and expands your range of motion in any posture. Resistance training increases muscular endurance and enables you to be comfortable in a wider variety of positions. While people of all shapes, sizes, and levels of ability can enjoy strap-on sex, you will find that with conditioning, your concerns will shift more toward pleasure and away from being winded and cramped.

Likewise, keep plenty of water by your bed to stay hydrated without missing a beat. Avoid excess use of drugs or alcohol before strap-on sex. While one drink or a few hits of a joint may lower your inhibitions and put you in a warm and fuzzy frame of mind, overindulgence can impair your judgment and make it more likely that you will injure yourself or your partner. Alcohol and drug use can dull pain. Pain during strap-on sex is a warning sign that something is wrong; physical injury may result if it is ignored. Make it a priority to remain clear-headed and attuned to your and your partner's bodily responses. Drug use can also affect your endurance and make it difficult to finish something you have started. The same can be true for excessive eating. While a sumptuous meal is often a prelude to a magical night filled with other corporeal delights, too much of a good thing may leave you feeling sluggish, sleepy, and uncomfortable.

Handiwork

Before you begin strap-on sex with your partner, use your hands to explore your mate's anatomy, especially if sex with a dildo and harness is new to you, or you are with a new partner. By using your hands, you can learn about the length and breadth of your partner's vagina or anus and how these structures change as she becomes aroused. Make the time and space to really explore your partner's body, to get to know the structures of her anatomy, and to gauge her sensitivities.

Go slowly as you progress toward dildo penetration. At times it takes more sexual confidence to go gradually rather to speed through the process. Some people enjoy being penetrated only after they have experienced a high degree of stimulation all over their bodies or on their clitoris or penis, or after being entered first with a smaller, hand-held dildo or fingers. Make sure that the receptive partner has reached his requisite level of arousal before engaging in strap-on sex. Failing to do so may result in discomfort, which can both hamper the current act of intercourse and

Repetitive Strain Injury

Repetitive strain injuries, such as carpal tunnel syndrome, are the bane of many folks in modern-day industries. In their book, *Repetitive Strain Injury*, Emil Pascarelli and Deborah Quilter describe the malady this way:

Fine hand movements, repeated hour after hour, day after day, thousands upon thousands of times, eventually strain the muscles and tendons of the forearms, wrists, and fingers, causing microscopic tears. Injured muscles tend to contract, decreasing the range of motion necessary for stress-free work. The sheaths that cover delicate tendons run out of lubrication because they aren't given time to rest, so tendons and sheath chafe. Now the insulted tissues become painful. In addition, there can be numbness, tingling, or hypersensitivity to touch.

As you may have suspected, strap-on sex can be a real boon to folks who have difficulties using their hands for vaginal or anal penetration. If you have a related injury, check out Everest and Jennings Avenues in the resources section at the back of the book. They offer a catalog full of adaptive devices for use with sexual toys, such as spandex mitts for holding small vibrators. Also, if you have hand, wrist or arm ailments and are using your hands in preparation for strap-on sex, make sure to observe healthy protocol, such as taking breaks frequently and changing positions as you go.

negatively color those that follow. It is always better to err on the side of too much foreplay than not enough.

Conditioned Response

Many people who initially find intense vaginal or anal stimulation excruciating will crave that same level of stimulation later in the same encounter or during a subsequent event. Preferences may change with age, level of arousal, pregnancy, stage of the menstrual cycle, trust in a particular partner, and conditioned response.

A conditioned response can be thought of as a pathway established in the neural circuitry with repeated experience. These responses can develop in association with a specific sexual act or a particular partner—they let your body know that you are traversing familiar terrain and allow you to progress more quickly to a state of sexual readiness when associated cues are present. A conditioned response can be compared with finding your way to a friend's house. On the first few visits you may need road maps and directions, but eventually you are able to reach your destination unaided. And so it is with sex—the more trust, warmth, and arousal is associated with a specific sexual act or partner, the more readily your body will respond to that act or person in the future.

Visualization

As you begin to penetrate your partner, keep in mind an image of the C curve of her vagina or the S curve of her anus. Be mindful of how these curves shift as your partner changes position. What happens to the S curve when your partner is on his back? How does it change when he raises one leg or puts his ankles on your shoulders? Where is her G-spot in relation to the tip of your dildo when she is on all fours? How does its position change when she arches her back? How must the curve of your dildo change to accommodate the arch of her rectum as she bends over a chair or sits on your lap?

A helpful hint for receptive partners: keep your hips above your head, regardless of your position. When your hips are elevated above your head, your vagina or anus is arrayed in front of your partner and she will have more control. When your head is higher than your hips, your pelvic region tilts backward. At this angle, the insertive partner has less ability to control the intensity and angle of stimulation, and the dildo will likely point sharply downward toward the receptive partner's perineum, pushing against the flesh and compressing it against her spine. This, let me say, is an experience best avoided.

While the mechanical aspects of angle and anatomy are vital to gratifying strap-on sex, it is also important to make the toy feel "real" enough for both partners. The more a strapper can project her sense of touch into a piece of silicone or mystery rubber, the more adept she will be at directing its motion and bringing pleasure to herself and her partner. Ultimately, however, the physical and emotional limits of the receptive partner must determine the parameters of the action.

The Five Variables

Should you encounter ergonomic difficulties during strap-on sex, evaluate the role of the following five basic factors to determine the source of the problem. Pay attention to how each of these factors operates in the positions you choose and experiment with manipulating these variables to enhance the satisfaction of you and your partner.

1. Adjust the height of the strapper. You can increase the height at which your dildo enters your mate by bringing her feet or knees together, by standing above her while she lies down, or by kneeling rather than

lying horizontally. To decrease your relative height, spread her feet or knees farther apart, or try sitting or reclining while your partner stands above you.

2. Adjust the height of the receptive partner. As you are being penetrated, you can lean over a chair, or you can place your feet flat on the surface upon which you are lying to change the level of your hips. Use a sling rather than a bed to increase the height of your vagina or anus. Push your legs further apart so that your vagina and anus are low and easier for a shorter partner to reach.

3. Adjust the angle of the strapper's body in relation to the receptive partner. As you penetrate your partner, prop yourself up with your hands so that you enter him at a more perpendicular angle, which will let you thrust more deeply. Lie directly on top of your partner and shift some of your weight to your forearms and knees to enable rapid thrusting. Or sit straight up with your partner on your lap for a full embrace during intercourse.

4. Adjust the angle of the receptive partner's body in relation to the strapper. As you are being penetrated, arch your back or prop your hips up on a pillow to make your vaginal or anal canal angle upward for easier access. Put your ankles on your partner's shoulders to situate your G-spot for intense stimulation. As the insertive partner, try holding your mate's hands behind her back so that her face is on the bed and her rectum bends down to match the curve of your dildo.

5. Adjust the length or angle of the dildo. An extra bit of dildo length can make certain positions easier to

achieve, but too much will prevent either partner from thrusting with full abandon. Dildo angle is critical in strap-on sex, and can be manipulated according to the requirements of the situation. For example, if you are penetrating your partner in the missionary position using a dildo with a slight upward angle, let the dildo jut from your pelvis unaided to provide indirect stimulation. To provide more intense stimulation later in the encounter, adjust the angle of the dildo by propping it up with the elastic band of your underwear. In other circumstances you may need to change toys or flip the one you are using upside down so that it points downward rather than upward; the latter technique is particularly useful when penetrating your partner from behind.

Come See About Me: Tips for Self-Stimulation

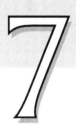

Many students who attend my advanced Strap-On Sex class have been humping away merrily for years, yet plunk down their twenty-five dollars just to have one question answered: "This strap-on stuff is all well and good, but how do *I* get off?" While many strappers find strap-on sex sufficiently pleasurable without specific physical stimulation, others want to find out how they can receive direct genital stimulation during strap-on sex. For these people, melding the emotional and fantasy elements of dildo and harness use with the experience of their physical body necessitates tools and techniques designed to provide the harness-wearer with stimulation during strap-on sex.

Thus strappers can be generally classified into three groups. The first consists of those for whom the emotional experience of strap-on sex alone is sufficiently satisfying. The second group is comprised of those for whom the contact provided by strap-on sex itself—the friction on the clitoris as it rubs against the base of the dildo or the repetitive movement of the crura and engorged tissue of the pelvic region—is adequate stimulus, and often brings them to orgasm. The final group consists of strappers who wish to augment the incidental friction of strap-on sex with other techniques to help them reach orgasm.

For the latter group, there are methods aplenty, ranging from the ingenious to the precarious. All are designed to enhance the experience of the harness-wearer during strap-on sex by providing her with some form of genital stimulation. The choice of technique depends both on the body parts the strapper wants to stimulate and the accoutrements with which he or she feels most comfortable. Female strappers can experiment with vaginal, clitoral, or anal stimulation, while male strappers may enhance strap-on sex through the use of toys and procedures that provide penis, anus, or prostate stimulation.

Clitoral Stimulation

Harnesses can easily be adapted for clitoral stimulation. Some women achieve sufficient clitoral pleasure by positioning the flange of their dildo so that it brushes against their clit as they thrust into their partner or by rubbing their clit up against the center strap of a thong-style harness. Others use one of the clever products on the market designed to provide clitoral stimulation during strap-on sex. These devices include the Leather Butterfly (from Stormy Leather), which is a pouch that holds a vibrating egg, such as the Silver Bullet or Pink Pearl, against the a strapper's clit, and the Magic Carpet (from Dills for Does), which is a textured silicone flap that strappers can position behind the flange of their dildo.

Ten Clitoral Stimulation Tips for Strappers

- Rub your clit against the center strap of a thong-style harness.
- Wear a Treasure Chest harness equipped with a bullet vibrator to provide clitoral stimulation for both yourself and your partner.
- Wrap a Stormy Leather vibro cuff around the center strap of a thong-style harness to hold a vibrating egg against your clitoris.
- Place a textured Magic Carpet inside the harness rig against the base of your dildo.
- Place a vibrating cock ring around the shaft of your dildo, turn the ring upside down, and tuck it behind your harness.
- Press the flange of a vibrating dildo against your clitoris to magnify friction.
- Use a dildo with nubs molded into the back of the flange and position it to stimulate your clit.
- Pump your clitoris to intensify stimulation while you penetrate your partner (see Chapter 9, All Pumped Up: Clit Pumping).
- Wear a Leather Butterfly pouch behind your harness to hold a vibrating egg against your clitoris.
- Use the pounding action of penetration to manipulate the crura of your clitoris as you thrust into your partner.

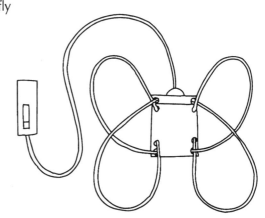

Illustration #7: Stormy Leather® Leather Butterfly

Vaginal Stimulation

Many people purchase a double-headed dildo, place it between themselves and their partner, and expect it to magically transform their bedroom into a chamber of carnal delights. With all due respect to the fine double-headed dildos available, this rarely happens. These toys require a great deal of dexterity and coordination, and one partner must have the presence of mind to hold on to it while pursuing nirvana. What's the solution then for couples bent on getting plenty of bang for both bodies during strap-on sex? Harness cuffs! That's right, whether the cuff is fixed to the front panel of a harness or attached with Velcro to the center strap, these accessories, which are designed to hold a dildo inside the harness-wearer, provide a more stable alternative for couples interested in doubling their vaginal or anal pleasure.

Cuffs are particularly advantageous in a number of situations. Perhaps you enjoy vaginal stimulation but prefer to avoid the sexual and gender dynamics of being penetrated by a partner. A dildo held in a cuff can provide a fair amount of vaginal stimulation for the harness-wearer, yet allows her to control the circumstances in which vaginal stimulation occurs. Other cuff users simply appreciate the convenience of dual penetration or incorporate cuff use while packing to hold a dildo inside themselves while on a date, at work, or writing how-to books.

Perhaps you enjoy vaginal stimulation during strap-on sex, but prefer that your partner penetrate you with his fingers or a hand-held dildo or vibrator as you fuck him with a strap-on. This maneuver requires a fair bit of skill and flexibility. If the receptive partner's arms are long enough, he can reach around his mate's back and beneath her ass to stimulate her vagina. Or he can place his hands through his partner's legs and stimulate her vagina underneath her strap-on rig. This is ideally performed with a jockstrap-style harness, which leaves the wearer's vulva available to her partner's caresses; when using a thong-style harness, the wearer or her partner can simply hold the center strap to one side.

Ten Vaginal Stimulation Tips for Strappers

- Use a fixed cuff, such as that on a Tuxedo thong-style harness, to hold a dildo inside your vagina.
- Use a silicone Magic Carpet clitoral/labial stimulator behind your dildo and harness to stimulate your entire vulva.
- Have your partner penetrate your vagina while you are wearing a jockstrap-style harness.
- Use a movable cuff with a thong-style harness to hold a dildo inside your vagina.
- Use two thigh harnesses to allow both partners to act as insertive and receptive partners simultaneously.
- Use a fixed or moveable cuff to hold a vibrating dildo inside your vagina.
- Use a dildo or vibrator to masturbate as your partner gives you a blow job.
- Have your partner use a hand-held dildo or vibrator to penetrate your vagina as you penetrate him with a dildo attached to a thigh harness.
- Hold a set of Duotone balls—hollow balls, made of plastic or silicone, with smaller balls inside them— inside your vagina as you penetrate your partner.
- Use a two-pronged dildo or vibrator to stimulate your vagina and anus simultaneously as you penetrate your partner.

Penile Stimulation

So strap-on sex sounds like fun to you boys, but you'd like to invite Mr. Willy to the party? There are a variety of ways to achieve penile stimulation while having an ever-ready auxiliary erection—or two—at your beck and call. Using a thigh harness creates ample opportunities for penis stimulation, since your dick is completely unobstructed. If you would like to involve your penis in strap-on sex but don't have an erection, slip a PPA—a hollow prosthetic device—over your flaccid penis. If you are already sporting a boner, you can use a harness to double your fun, by strapping on a dildo above your factory-equipped penis and penetrating your partner's vagina and anus simultaneously.

Ten Penile Stimulation Tips for Strappers

- Have your partner stroke your penis as you penetrate him with a dildo in a thigh harness.
- Jerk off as you penetrate your partner with a thigh-mounted dildo.
- Use a penis pump to provide stimulation as you penetrate your partner with a dildo in a thigh harness.
- Wear a vibrating cock ring around your penis while using a dildo strapped to your pubic mound to penetrate your partner.
- Wear a vibrating sleeve over your penis while you penetrate your partner with a dildo strapped to your pubic mound.
- Place your erect penis beneath the harness and rub your penis against your partner's abdomen or ass as you penetrate him with a dildo.
- If you are a female-to-male transgendered person, insert your neophallus into a plastic clit-pumping cylinder fitted with a Cyberskin sheath with a three-inch extension; use this to penetrate your partner.

- Inserts your flaccid penis into a PPA held around your hips by elastic bands; use this to penetrate your partner.
- Strap a dildo and harness to your pubic mound above your erect penis; in the missionary position, penetrate your partner's vagina with the dildo and her anus with your penis.
- Using a thigh harness, hold your partner on your lap, dildo inside him, as you or he strokes your penis.

Anal Stimulation

Many strappers, both male and female, enjoy anal stimulation during strap-on sex. A butt plug, for example, is specifically designed to provide a no-hands alternative for anal eroticism. A well-made medium or large size anal plug can function independently of a harness, while dildos and smaller anal plugs can be held in the strapper's ass using a movable cuff fastened to the center strap of a thong-style harness. See Chapter 10, Anal Exploits, for more on toys for anal play.

Some strappers enjoy anal penetration literally at the hands of their partners, who can reach behind them

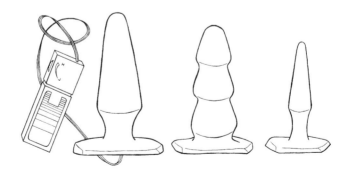

Illustration #8: Butt plugs

with a dildo or their fingers during strap-on sex. This is most easily done when the strapper is wearing a jockstrap-style harness, which leaves the anus unobstructed. Other strappers crave vibration against their anus, which can be accomplished using a vibro cuff, a leather pouch that snaps around the center strap of a thong-style harness and holds a vibrating egg against the strapper's anus.

Ten Anal Stimulation Tips for Strappers

- Use a butt plug for hands-free anal stimulation.
- Use a movable cuff attached to a thong-style harness to hold a dildo in your anus.
- Have your partner penetrate your anus with her fingers or a dildo as you penetrate her with a dildo mounted in a jockstrap-style harness.
- Use a harness to hold a plug or dildo in your anus while you penetrate your partner with a dildo mounted in a thigh harness.
- Use a vibro pouch attached to the center strap of a thong-style harness to hold a vibrating egg against your anus.
- Have your partner hold a Hitachi Magic Wand with a penetrating attachment against your anus.
- Have your partner penetrate your anus with her fingers or a hand-held dildo while you penetrate her with a dildo in thigh harness.
- Use a moveable cuff attached to a thong-style harness to hold a vibrating butt plug in your anus.
- Insert a string of silicone anal beads, which can be pulled out at an auspicious moment as you penetrate your partner.
- Use a vibro pouch to hold a bullet vibrator against your clitoris, a fixed cuff to hold a dildo inside your vagina, and a movable cuff to hold a butt plug in your anus.

Dear Fairy Butch,

My mind tends to work in the strangest ways. Please tell me,
how many sex toys can you use at one time, seriously?

—Inquiring Mind

Dear Inquiring:

Kumquat, fear not! Your very own Fairy Butch has had the
very same concern for neigh on twenty-two years. Imagine if you
will, a little baby Fairy Butch, ensconced in the bosom of America
that is Dayton, Ohio, spending fervent afternoons with a box of
chocolate Kraft food sticks and a mind filled with prurient imagin-
ings. I fancied myself a sexually-obsessed scientist in a remote
mansion. I spent my days designing spinning, multi-pronged
instruments of pleasure, and my nights employing them on
gorgeous, buxom vixens awaiting my ministrations. Ah, youth.

But I digress. There is no definitive limit that one can use at
any one time, Pet! Let your imagination run wild! Perhaps you
could strap on a dildo, while wearing a dildo in your pussy, a
butt plug in your ass, and a vibrator in a pouch attached to your
harness, over you clit. Whilst you work the dildo in your lover's
(or trick's, as the case may be) cooch, you could have another
butt plug in her tush, while she holds a Hitachi magic wand on
her clit. She might be restrained via both ankle and wrist
restraints, and you could use one hand to hold on to her via a
collar, leash, and a Y-chain attached to both her nipples and clit,
and the other to treat her back to a good lashing featuring a
cowhide whip.

Let's see, that's 13, but I'm certain that folks in my little
audience have their own thoughts regarding taking toys to the
max. Send' em my way, Pumpkin, and we'll compare notes!
XOXOXOXO,
Fairy Butch

Packing: Taking Your Show on the Road

Imagine you're in the back of a darkened movie theater with your arm around your date, sexual tension crackling in the air. You reach over to kiss the back of her neck. She moves her hand to your knee, and you grasp it and bring it up along your thigh to the hard bulge beneath your jeans. All at once your intentions are made clear. That's right, you're packing.

Packing is simply the act of wearing a dildo underneath one's clothing—a rigid member for hard packing, or a more malleable device for packing soft. The significance of packing, however, is far more complex. Hard packing refers to wearing a dildo and harness rig with the intention of later using it for strap-on sex. When you pack hard, you signal a variety of intentions to your partner. First, you convey that you were thinking about sex before even leaving the house, and that you were perhaps in a state of sexual arousal as you suited up. Second, you indicate that your sexual interests include penetration. Finally, you show that you are prepared to take action on the fly and in a variety of locations.

Soft packing involves the use of a pliant device, or a harness and flexible dildo, to convey the feel and appearance of a penis and scrotum in repose, rather than standing at attention.

> If I'm not packing a hard-on that's ready to use, I incorporate my need to go "get ready" with the mood. I usually give explicit orders of some sort that allow me the few minutes I need to suit up.

> I like my cock to be real-looking, so I pack with what I hope I will be using.

> I love, let me say that again...love when my butch packs. In fact, the mere topic of packing makes me... well...never mind...

Hard Packing

If you are going out for a night on the town and you want to be ready for all possibilities, come what may, get set to pack for action. Although genderplay is often a feature of packing for action, if you want to penetrate your partner in a fun, no-fumble fashion, regardless of your gender identity or fantasy, you are a candidate for hard packing. If you're worried that packing an erect dildo will make you look like a kangaroo carrying her young, fear not. With some consideration and a few accessories, you can create a manageable bulge that will attract the attention only of those in the market for your goods.

You can pack a dildo in a variety of ways; the method you choose may be inspired by the type of dildo you're packing, the evening's ensemble, or several other factors. Your packing technique can become a part of the sexual act itself if you use the elastic of your underwear to hoist up your dick during sex or if your clothing itself acts as a harness, as with the case of the Levi's 501 pack. When considering packing efficacy and comfort, evaluate the dildo you have selected, the amount of time you will be wearing the rig, how much of a bulge you want to show, and when and where you plan to penetrate your partner. Experiment with some of the techniques listed below to find a system that works best for your specific needs.

The Jockstrap Pack

To execute the jockstrap pack, select a harness and a dildo with a flange. Assemble them so that the straps on one side of the harness are fastened and the other side is left free. Step through the strap-on rig with one leg, and adjust the straps evenly around your body. Keep the harness loosely fastened so that the dildo is not fully erect underneath your clothes. You may wish to wear a pair of underwear underneath the harness and dildo to protect your pubic mound from friction against the flange. Turn the dildo so that it points to one side under the fold of your belly to facilitate a tighter pack against your body.

Stuff the dildo into a sturdy jockstrap with a firm elastic band. Slip the tip of the toy underneath the elastic band for an even tighter pack. Femme packers may choose to substitute a more frilly yet substantial undergarment. Slip the whole package into a snug pair of boxers, preferably the button variety, with a firm elastic waistband.

Just prior to sexual contact, tighten up the harness rig and adjust the dildo so that it is in an erect position against your pubic mound. During sex you can either use the elastic waistbands from both the jockstrap and the boxers to hoist the dildo up, or use the elastic from the jockstrap to support the dick from underneath and feed it through the unbuttoned fly of the boxers. The latter method lets you hide the entire harness rig, with only the dildo visible.

The Tuxedo Pack

The Tuxedo pack requires a Tuxedo harness, a model equipped with an attached cuff designed to hold a dildo inside the vagina of a female harness wearer, and a dildo with a flange. Alternatively, a detached cuff can be used with other types of harness. Assemble the dildo and harness so that one side is fastened together and the other side is left free. Step through the harness rig with one leg and adjust the straps evenly around your body. Keep the harness loosely fastened to facilitate a comfortable fit underneath your clothes. You may want to wear a pair of underwear beneath the harness and dildo to protect your pubic mound from friction against the flange. The Tuxedo pack works well with most types of apparel, so feel free to don skirts or tight jeans. When using a Tuxedo harness, turn the dildo around so that it curves downward, feed it through the fixed cuff between your legs, and snap or Velcro it into place. When using a harness other than the Tuxedo model, turn the dildo around so that it curves downward and wrap the cuff around both the tip of the dildo and the center strap of a thong-style harness. If you are using a jockstrap-style harness, wrap the cuff around one of the side straps. Snap or Velcro the cuff into place.

Just prior to sexual contact, tighten up the harness rig and adjust the dildo so that it is an erect position against your pubic mound.

The Levi's 501 Pack

Another popular packing technique requires a pair of Levi's 501 or similar button-fly jeans snug enough so that the crotch is taut across your pubic mound. Select any dildo with a flange. Don't worry about a harness—you're already wearing it! This method is great if you cannot afford a harness or do not have one available at the moment.

The 501 pack works best if you wear thick, snug underwear such as men's jockeys or boxers underneath your jeans. Place the dildo in your underwear, either pointing up and to one side underneath the fold of your belly, or between your legs if you can stand the prolonged genital stimulation. You may wish to wear an additional pair of underwear underneath the dildo, to protect your pubic mound from friction against the flange, and a third pair over the dildo for a smoother appearance.

During strap-on sex, fasten the top and bottom buttons of the jeans, and use the remaining buttons to hold the dildo firmly in place at a desirable angle. Make certain the flange of the dildo is tightly secured by the material of the jeans. Button-fly boxers can be helpful because you can keep the top button undone and use the bottom button to help support the weight of the dildo behind the jeans.

Soft Packing

Soft packing, or packing as a gender signifier, is intended to create the appearance of a soft or semi-hard penis and scrotum underneath your clothing. The aim of soft packing is to convey the appearance of a male package, rather than to prepare for actual intercourse. Because soft packing is generally more comfortable and subtle than hard packing, there are a variety of scenarios which might lead you to choose it over the harder variety. Drag kings—women who depict men for theatrical or camp value—often pack soft in order to portray a realistic representation of their characters. Likewise, many female-to-male transsexuals pack soft on a daily basis to present a natural-looking crotch as they go about their affairs. You may choose to pack soft and carry a strap-on rig with a firmer dildo to change into later for strap-on sex

> I really enjoy when my boyfriend packs. I find it highly sexy. There is a little something different about his attitude when he does...he seems more powerful.

> When I pack a hard-on, the jock strap helps the chafing. And my buckling leg harness keeps the dildo from traveling all over the place. You have to choose whether you are going to dress right or left, and certain pants feel better than others. I have a dildo with a slight angle that I wear upside down so it curves in toward my leg, not up toward the moon.

The Packing Device Pack

The packing device pack method involves the use of a dildo designed solely for the purpose of creating the appearance of a soft penis and testicles underneath full dress, swim trunks, or underwear. When using a prosthetic soft cock-and-balls combo such as the Bulge, the Ingersoll, the Packer, or the Ultimate Packer, simply place the device in a snug pair of jockeys so that it resembles a soft penis and testicles. Wear any type of clothing you like over the underwear.

The Hair Gel, Condom, and Stocking Pack

The hair gel, condom, and stocking is great if you want to create the appearance of a soft penis and testicles, but you have more time on your hands than money. This technique uses inexpensive, easily attainable materials to create a soft package underneath full dress, swim trunks, or underwear.

Gather six non-lubricated condoms and a tube of unscented, alcohol-free hair gel. Some packers prefer to use a children's product called Gak that can be found in most toy stores. Experiment with both and see which kind of squish you prefer. Squeeze the gel into a condom until it is about half full. Form the gel into a teardrop shape by tying the empty part of the condom off at the top. Double-bag this package with another condom, and place it in a knee-high stocking for extra protection and firmness. This will be the first testicle. Repeat the above steps to create the second testicle, and tie the two testicles together with the excess stocking material at the top of the package.

Fill another condom with gel to form the penis, tie off the top, and place it into another knee-high stocking. Fasten it to the balls with the excess stocking material. Place the entire package in a snug pair of jockeys so that it resembles a soft penis and testicles and wear any type of clothing you like over the underwear. This creation should last up to six months; be sure to replace it after this amount of time so that it doesn't break at an inauspicious moment.

> Most days I pack flaccid using a homemade pants stuffer made from condoms and Gak and an old pair of nylons. This all is pinned into my shorts and fills out my pants. It doesn't look like I have a piece of firewood shoved down my pants, and it's comfortable.

The Pack 'n' Play Pack

For more versatile soft packing, use a Pack 'n' Play dildo made by Vixen Creations, or any other dildo that is designed to give a semi-hard appearance underneath clothing and that converts to a functional sex toy by turning it upside down. For simple soft packing, stash the Pack 'n' Play in a snug pair of jockeys or briefs so that it resembles a semi-erect penis and testicles. Wear any type of clothing you like over the underwear.

If you plan to use the dildo for strap-on sex, wear a harness with the toy. Thong-style harnesses work better than jockstrap-style models for this type of device. Strap the dildo and harness loosely to your body so that its position approximates that of a semi-erect penis and testicles. Wear a snug pair of underwear over the rig. When you are ready to use the toy for sex, simply remove it from the harness, flip it upside down so it points upward, reinsert it into the harness, and tighten the harness straps around your body. This toy works well for intense G-spot or prostate stimulation when the receptive partner is on her or his back. If the receptive partner is on hands and knees, try leaving the Pack 'n' Play pointing downward.

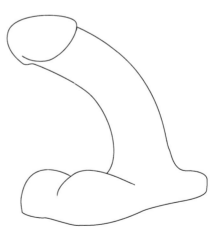

Illustration #9: Vixen Pack 'n' Play

Dear Fairy Butch,

I am a kind of femme girl, and one of the things I have always wanted to do is pack a big dildo as a special surprise when I take someone home (or rather, get someone to take me home.) But I don't want to step on anybody's toes. I know
some women have issues about this sort of thing. Is it wrong to pull this kind of surprise? I don't want to misrepresent my gender/sexuality to anyone. Also, is it bad manners to use the same toy on a variety of women?

—Pretty and Packing

Dear Pretty:

You go, girl! I'm sure that there are many butches who would love to find such a treasure lurking beneath your smart skirt. Banish those gender prescriptions and work that rod to your heart's content! That's the wonderful thing about being a modern-day dyke: you get to make it up as you go along. Keep what works for you, sister, and discard the rest.

As for the butch ego, it can indeed be a fragile thing. But much of this is due to a perceived expectation that we must always wear the pants (or, in this case, the dick). The next time you spy the stud girl of your dreams leaning up against the bar, Budweiser in hand, saunter over and snatch a bit of control for yourself. Set the tone: ask her to dance, have the bartender bring her a cold beer. As the intensity mounts, push back if she presses you into a darkened corner, tug at her hair, and by all means, let your packed panties press into her denimed crotch.

If she's still with you at this point, then chances are she'll think she's found Nirvana; she might just be thrilled to have the tables turned on her. Live your dreams, Sugar. Work up that sexy femme confidence, strap on that dildo, and I'll wager that before long, a coterie of butches will beat a path to your door, toes pointed north, and legs accommodatingly spread wide open.

If, however, you intend to use the same dildo on each and every one of these lucky gals, you'll have to take some precautions. If you elect to use a non-silicone specimen, use a condom on it each and every time. These toys can be very porous, and though they can be cleaned with antibacterial soap and warm water, they cannot be disinfected. Make your partner her get on her hands and knees and slip the condom on with her mouth, if you like, but make sure you're covered.

If you decide to employ a silicone dick in your adventure, then you have a bit more latitude in the situation, as long as you properly disinfect the toy by boiling it in water or placing it in the top rack of your dishwasher between uses. Nonetheless, I still encourage you to glove your love in case your partner becomes so enthralled with your technique that she wants it up her ass, or alternatively, wants to do an about-face in your direction. In either case, it is important that you have a disinfected dick, and odds are that running a load of dishes won't be the foremost thing on your mind. Simply pull off the used condom, roll on a new one, and you're ready to go.

XOXOXOXO,

Fairy Butch

The Bait and Switch

Like the Pack 'n' Play pack, the bait and switch method also combines soft and hard packing. However, instead of packing an all-in-one toy, you pack soft and carry a harness rig with a firmer dildo to put on later for strap-on sex. To set the bait, pack either a prosthetic soft cock-

and-balls combination such as the Bulge, the Ingersoll, the Packer, or the Ultimate Packer, or a homemade gel, condom, and stocking package. You may also use a smaller, softer dildo than the one you will use later for intercourse. If using a prosthetic packer alone, place the device in a snug pair of jockeys so that it resembles a soft penis and testicles. Wear any type of clothing you like over the underwear. You can stash both the firm dildo and a harness in a toy bag or coat pocket, or you can wear the harness underneath your soft packer and store just the dildo.

If you choose to use two dildos for this method, strap the smaller, softer dildo into a harness of your choice and assemble it so that one side is fastened and the other side is left free. Step through the harness with one leg and adjust the straps evenly around your body. Keep the harness loosely fastened so that the dildo is not fully erect underneath your clothes. A dildo made of a softer material such as Cyberskin or PVC will give you a definite phallic bulge beneath your clothing, but is more comfortable to pack than a larger toy made of a denser materials such as silicone.

When you are ready for strap-on sex, slip into a bathroom with the sack or jacket containing your harness and firm dildo. You can suit up quickly when wearing pants by pulling down your trousers, unfastening the harness on both sides, slipping it through your legs over your underwear, and refastening the straps. If you are already wearing a harness, simply remove the soft dildo and replace it with the firmer one. Arrange the dildo in an erect position, tighten up the harness straps so that it is comfortable but snug, and pull your trousers up.

All Pumped up: Clit Pumping

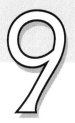

Odds are that even if you are a well-seasoned sexual adventurer, you will find novelty in the notion of having your clit pumped up to many times its normal size—just imagine what you or your partner could do with the extra real estate. I first contemplated the possibilities of clit pumping some years ago when a boy's toys section was added to Good Vibrations. I was in school then and the pressure of scholarly procrastination fueled my sexual imagination to dizzying new heights. I scanned the shelves full of handsome new black, rubber dick vibrators and studded cock rings, looking for a new method to apply to my sexual madness, until at last, I found it—the lucite San Francisco Pumpworks cylinders and accompanying brass hand pump. Men use these items to create a vacuum seal around the base of the penis; pumping out the air causes the penis to swell with blood, making it considerably larger and more sensitive.

Along with the penis-sized cylinders, I found considerably smaller cylinders designed to work their pneumatic magic on nipples. As I experimented with the intense sucking action of these tubes on the skin on the back of my hand, I wondered how the same pressure might feel directed about two feet lower—between my legs. Finally, I coughed up the cash and procured a system for myself. I took the apparatus home and set about creating my own phallus—or at least making something new, exciting, and larger out of the genital tissue nature had provided me. I scoured gay men's toy stores for a means to extend my experience—and my clitoris—beyond the dimensions of a small nipple cylinder. Much to my delight, I found many fascinating products, none of which were designed to fuel the fire of female loins, but which nonetheless could be adapted to do that very thing.

Soon I found myself amidst piles of pumps and foreskin cylinders, thin cock rings designed after bolo ties, finger cots, Vaseline tins, razors and the like. I decided to share my discovery with the participants in my advanced Strap-On Sex class and began teaching others the methods I had developed. I soon discovered that female-to-male transsexuals had been pumping up for years. Like the wheel, clit pumping had been invented independently in different places and at different times.

While clit pumping is not for everyone, it can be enjoyed by anyone with a yen for sexual adventure, an awareness of safety, and access to the requisite equipment. The process lends itself particularly well to gender-bending fantasies, as the effect of possessing genitals the size of a small penis can be a boon to female-bodied individuals who aspire to a more manly aspect, either temporarily or permanently. Yet clit pumping need not imply masculinization if that does not suit your sexual purposes. Whether you are transgendered, stone butch, or a gal looking for a new way to expand her horizons, clit pumping can provide a wonderful new way to enhance your sexuality.

Safety Precautions

Clit pumping is a sophisticated procedure, and you should attempt it only if you are willing to apply great care and attention to your body and its responses. The process requires a significant time commitment and should be done in a relaxed atmosphere without time constraints. Feel free to take long breaks from pumping to adapt to the sensation of the vacuum as your clit grows. Proceed with caution, avoid the use of intoxicants, and halt immediately if you feel pain. Unlike S/M activities, such as whipping and paddling, *pain during clit pumping is a definite signal to stop*. Though there may be microscopic tearing of the mucous membranes with any form of genital sex, pain is indicative of too much tearing too fast. Stop.

Likewise, do not try clit pumping if there are any bruises or lesions on your genitals or if you have any infections or diseases. There has been no scientific research on clit pumping—in fact, there isn't even much anecdotal data about the practice. While clit pumping has brought pleasure to many of its devotees and their partners, it is a delicate and time-consuming process that could cause injury if done incorrectly.

Why Clit Pumping?

Why would a person be interested in pumping her clit? For many people, the first question that comes to mind is whether a pumped-up clitoris can be used for penetration. The answer is yes, but with several caveats. Some experienced practitioners have pumped their clits to 4 $\frac{1}{2}$

inches in length and 5 inches around (while still in the cylinder). Indeed, they have been able to insert their appendage into their partner. A pumped clitoris doesn't resemble an erect penis, and is, in fact, more akin to a flaccid dick.

A major benefit of clit pumping is the imagery it offers. It can be validating to have your genitals look more like what people generally think of as male, if that's the effect you are trying to achieve. Clit pumping can also offer a rewarding visual experience for your partner, who may never view your genitals in quite the same way. Finally, clit pumping can just be kinky fun.

But let's not put the cart before the horse—the pumping process provides its own pleasures independent of how the final result is utilized. The term *clit pumping* is actually a misnomer. In addition to the clitoris, the clitoral hood and the surrounding labia minora are also often involved in the pumping process. As you pump, the clitoris typically retracts under its hood and becomes harder. The hood moves forward to cover the clitoral glans and swells with blood and other fluids, profoundly accelerating the natural course of vasocongestion, the process by which the body naturally prepares itself for sexual activity. Clit pumping can thus be a neat trick for jump-starting your libido. As your body makes the connection between the swelling of your genitals and sexual arousal, your own particular sexual response cycle will likely come into play. The genital tissues stretch during clit pumping and may become extremely sensitive and delicate. Be sure to treat them with care.

As a clit pumper, it is important to develop the patience to appreciate the journey as well as the destination. Pace yourself when you pump—go slowly, allow your body to accommodate the growth, and then, if desired, pump some more. Clit pumping is a very subjective experience. Some people report that the pump feels like intense oral sex, while others have a difficult time likening the sensation to anything else they have experienced. Some pumpers achieve orgasm from the sucking sensation alone, while others enjoy the intensity of the sensation without orgasm. Some pumping aficionados enjoy the process as a stand-alone thrill, while others prefer to include it as one part of a combination of sexual activities. Clit pumping can be readily integrated with strap-on sex, oral sex, and clitoral, vaginal, or anal stimulation. Finally, some people try clit pumping and find that it's not for them.

Clit pumping practitioners vary in the degree of pumping they pursue. Some want only a tiny amount of clitoral suction, while other seek a modest bit of temporary clitoral and labial growth. Still others attempt to stretch the limits of the endeavor as far as they can be taken. Those who enjoy a lesser degree of suction can loosen the nipple cylinder valve to allow air flow and prevent the creation of a vacuum hold. The sucking action is still in force in this variation, but because there is no adherence between the cylinder and the genitals, the tissue does not swell. Those who seek moderate, temporary genital growth can close the valve on the nipple cylinder to create a vacuum. Those who want to go for broke can use a foreskin cylinder to allow the clitoris to reach its maximum potential.

Toys for Beginners

If you'd like to wade into the clit pumping waters gradually, there are a few toys on the market that provide an excellent introduction to the concept of pumping, yet require a lesser financial and physical commitment. The first is the snakebite kit, which contains two yellow rubber suction cups, a scalpel, and snake venom antidote. Once you've tossed the contents of the rubber suckers (or have used them up saving the life of poor snakebite victim), lubricate one of the suckers, squeeze it together around the flesh of your clitoris, and let go. The sucker will stay in place until you squeeze it together again and break the suction.

Similar devices designed for sexual use, such as the Black Suckerfish, are available from Adam and Gillian's Sensual Whips and Toys. These attractive, heavy-duty suction cups are attached to one another with a chain. Many sex toy stores carry inexpensive generic black suction cups. Although these toys are much less intense than the vacuum methods that follow, you should still practice caution and common sense when using them. Do not leave the suction cups on your genitals for more than a few minutes at first.

A Proffering of Pumps

First you must select your pumping system from the two basic systems available. For the sake of clarity, I will refer to these as the cupping method and the hose-pump method. The former method utilizes a non-heating mechanical cupping set. Never try clit pumping with a heated cupping kit. Use only mechanical systems that achieve suction through the use of a squeeze pump. You can find these systems at some massage, sex, and fetish stores.

There are several advantages to the cupping method over the hose-pump method, including lower cost, convenience, comfort, and ease of use. First, a cupping kit comes complete with a well-made pump and cylinders of different sizes, all for about $80. Second, the cupping method is much easier to use than the hose-pump system. Because the cupping system is a solid unit, you need not concern yourself with a hose flopping around, and the apparatus can easily be held against your clitoris with one hand. Finally, because the cupping cylinders are flared at one end, and because the genital tissue is not stretched as intensely as with the hose-pump system, the cupping method is ideal for beginners and for those desiring a less intense effect. Since the suction is not as strong, there is less risk of injuring the genital tissue. The cupping method is also advantageous if you have a shorter period of time to devote to the project or if you want to plump up your genitals or enhance your libido in preparation for partner sex or masturbation. Cupping can also be used as a introductory phase to quickly warm up and increase blood flow to the genitals before moving on to the hose-pump system.

Nonetheless, the hose-pump system is the only way to achieve an intense suction effect and dramatically increase the size of your clitoris. Either a nipple or a foreskin cylinder can be attached to the hose-pump by means of a secure coupler valve. When the valve is closed and a tight seal has been made against the pumper's skin, no air can escape and a vacuum is created. Another advantage of the hose-pump system is that the cylinder can be detached from the pump, leaving the suction unaffected. Thus you can (gingerly) walk around or pursue other sexual activities while maintaining the clit pumping effect.

Clit Pumping and the Julia Child Aesthetic

When I was a child, I had a penchant for Julia Child's televised cooking classes and strove to imitate her sense of organization and panache in the kitchen. Julia always set out premeasured ingredients in an orderly and convenient fashion, devised a clean and comfortable work setting, and ensured that she had the proper tools available for every phase of the job. Likewise, before you embark on your clit pumping endeavor, select the equipment which best suits your needs, make certain that you have a suitable setting, and have all the necessary accoutrements gathered round you. At a minimum you will need the follow equipment:

- A pump system, snakebite kit, or mechanical cupping kit
- Vaseline
- baby oil
- shaving equipment
- paper towels
- access to warm water, preferably a shower or bath
- washcloths and towels
- any other toys you would like to use in conjunction with pumping.

Prime Your Pump

It is important that the flesh of your genitals be warm and engorged with blood to facilitate comfortable pumping. This may be accomplished by taking a steamy hot shower or applying warm washcloths to the genital area for ten to fifteen minutes—or masturbating! (Make sure that the shower isn't too long though—you don't want to feel faint prior to the process of pumping.) To achieve a tight seal when using the pump, shave the skin where the cylinder will make contact; the presence of pubic hair will break the seal required to create the vacuum effect. It is possible instead to merely trim the hair in this area, but you will not in achieve the same kind of adherence hairless skin provides. Shaving is less important when using the cupping system, which is not designed to create a tight seal.

Towel dry and apply a coat of Vaseline to the skin where the cylinder will make contact. Then coat the entire inside of the cylinder with baby oil to prevent friction between your genitals and the plastic. Be sure to coat the cylinder fully with oil. Drain any excess baby oil from the cylinder on some paper towels and attach it to the pump. If you plan to use a latex dental dam, condom, or other safer sex gear, remove the Vaseline and baby oil prior to the use of latex to prevent degrading the material. If you are sensitive to petroleum or oil-based products or are especially prone to vaginal infections, try substituting a thick, gel-type water-based lubricant such as Embrace or Maximus for the Vaseline, and a thin water-based lubricant such as Slippery Stuff Liquid for the baby oil. In any case, keep oil-based products out of your vagina.

Pumping in Repose: The Cupping System

A cupping system includes several different size plastic cylinders and a one-hand squeeze pump. Because there is no hose attached to the pump, it is easy to operate with one hand. Since the connection between the valve at the top of the cylinder and mouth of the pump is much weaker than with a hose-pump system, you will not experience a hard suction sensation on your clitoris and surrounding tissues. Nonetheless, take your time and listen to your body's responses. Experiment with using various cylinder sizes to encompass different amounts of genital flesh, and try using the pump at different angles.

Power Pumping: The Hose-Pump Method

There are two types of pumping devices available for use with a hose-pump system. One is the traditional brass hand pump, modeled after a bicycle pump. The other is a one-hand squeeze pump model equipped with an escape trigger on the handle, manufactured by companies such as Neward Enterprises. If you use the traditional pump, prop the brass part underneath your chin like a violin and pump with one hand while the other holds the cylinder against your groin. The traditional pump may be a better choice if you have carpal tunnel syndrome or a similar disorders, since the squeeze pump requires repetitive motions that can worsen these problems.

Once you have chosen your pump, attach the hose to the coupler valve on the end of the nipple cylinder; most nipple cylinders are 1 inch in diameter and about 4 inches long. Insert your clitoris and clitoral hood into the cylinder and establish a tight contact between the cylinder opening and the shaved skin at the base of the clitoral hood. The valve should be screwed in loosely at first to permit air to escape; this is important, since it can be dangerous to start heavy suction immediately. Your clitoris will extend into the cylinder when the pump is engaged, and will retreat back toward your pubic mound when the pump is released. If the valve is not tightened, the cylinder will not adhere to your skin; instead you will feel a rhythmic sucking as you pump, and your genitals will gradually become engorged. Many people limit their clit pumping to this initial stage. Those who desire to forge ahead should spend a significant amount of time here to prevent injury from too much suction, too soon.

If you venture beyond the initial stage, you will experience much more intense sucking sensations as you close the cylinder valve. When your clitoris and labia start to fill the cylinder, you can gradually tighten the valve. The more you turn the valve, the greater the suction power of the pump. As you tighten the valve, make certain that the pump hose is free of kinks or fissures and that the opening of the cylinder is held firmly against your skin to prevent air from escaping. Go slowly and pay careful attention to the signals your body is sending you. Stop pumping immediately if the process causes pain.

When the cylinder valve is fully closed, the vacuum pressure becomes especially intense; be careful not to pump too much. Once you have reached a comfortable level of suction, you can carefully disconnect the pump and go about your business. When the intense pulling sensation on your genitals lessens, pump a bit more and allow your body to rest again to safely accommodate the new growth. Do not get overzealous and start pumping for all you're worth; if you go too fast and go further than feels comfortable, your genitals could sustain damage and lose sensation. To release the valve with traditional pump, simply loosen the screw where the hose connects to the valve. With the squeeze pump, just pull on the release trigger to allow the air to escape. Be sure to familiarize yourself with these release mechanisms before you need to use them.

When your clit has comfortably filled the nipple cylinder, remove the cylinder, rest for a moment, and marvel at your gorgeous creation. Give your clit a rub, and warm it in your hands or the hands of a friend. If the tissue is cool, you'll want to wait until it is warm again before you proceed with pumping. Many folks stop at this point and enjoy the robust sensitivity the process has afforded them; others keep the nipple cylinder on as they pursue other sexual pastimes.

Should you be into more extreme sports, you can move on to a larger Plexiglas foreskin cylinder. These come in two sizes: 4 inches long by 5 inches around and 4 inches long by 6 inches around. Each foreskin cylinder comes with a small plastic ball and ring designed to stretch the foreskin and break adhesions between the foreskin and glans of a man's penis. For the purposes of clit pumping, you will need only the cylinder itself.

Before using the larger cylinder, reapply Vaseline to the skin around your genitals if necessary. Coat the inside of the larger cylinder with baby oil. Wipe up any excess oil or Vaseline that may have flowed toward the urethra or the opening of vaginal canal before carefully repeating the entire clit pumping procedure with the new cylinder.

Acclimate your genitals to the new cylinder by starting to pump with the valve open. There is no requisite period of time to pump with an open valve before you begin to tighten it; listen to your own body—let your body guide you as you gradually tighten the valve and increase the intensity of the suction.

Want Some Company, Honey?

Some people enjoy clit pumping best while in the company of a supportive and caring partner, while others prefer to do it on their own. In either case, it is important that the atmosphere be relaxed and free of pressure. You may wish to experiment and become comfortable with pumping on your own before you introduce it into the sexual repertoire you share with your partner. Partners are often eager to get their hands on your newly-fashioned goods, but some may initially be put off by the unknown. If this is the case, make sure to do your pumping alone first so that you can gain confidence in the procedure before you involve someone else. If you feel positive and happy about your pumped-up clit, your partner will likely follow suit.

Après Pumping

Many sexual activities can be more intense and pleasurable after you pump up your clitoris and remove the cylinder, especially since your libido will likely be amplified. Pressure of any kind will be magnified due to the amount of blood in the genital tissues. Even rubbing up against a partner with your swollen clit can feel especially good after pumping. Make certain though to completely remove any trace of Vaseline or baby oil before you proceed with genital stimulation.

Oral sex can be greatly intensified as well after pumping, and the effect of every suck, lick, and nuzzle may be greatly increased. In fact, pre-orgasmic or intermittently orgasmic women may be able to increase their potential for climax during oral sex. Some female-bodied people such as transmen and stone butches who do not identify with their female genitalia find that oral sex is transformed after clit pumping; because the size of the clitoris may increase dramatically, fantasies of fellatio are easily accommodated. Individuals who were formerly reluctant to allow their partners to perform oral sex on them may change their tune after pumping up.

A pumped clitoris can greatly the increase pleasurable sensations for either partner in strap-on sex, manual penetration, anal sex, and non-clitorally-focused sexual activities such as body stroking and kissing. Vibrators should be used cautiously on a freshly pumped clit since sensations will be greatly magnified. If your clitoris has been pumped large enough, you can experiment with a dick vibrator designed for smaller penises. Whichever sexual activity you pursue, you may wish to use a loose cord or a bolo cock ring to carefully restrict the flow of blood back out of your clitoris, helping it stay bigger and harder for a longer time. Use an extra small condom, a finger cot, or a dental dam or plastic food wrap to provide safer sex protection; be careful to thoroughly remove any oil-based products that could degrade latex.

If you prefer to keep the suction working for you while you play, simply detach the hose of a hose-pump system after pumping and leave the cylinder in place around your clit. Tugging lightly on the cylinder can be quite pleasurable, but do not tug too hard or you will to break the suction. If the cylinder does fall off, simply reapply Vaseline, insert your genitals back into the cylinder, and pump them up again. Try using a vibrator against the cylinder to intensify the effect of both devices. Spencer Bergstadt, a Seattle area FTM, recommends covering the cylinder with fabric to muffle the sound of a plastic vibrator moving against the plastic cylinder:

> It's lots of fun to jerk off with the cylinder on, yanking on it to pull the skin down over the corona of my little dick.

Keeping the cylinder on during strap-on sex requires a bit of finesse. Some thong-style harnesses have a hole in the leather front panel through which you can insert your cylinder-encased clitoris. If you are using a jockstrap-style harness, you may be able to accommodate the cylinder by pulling the harness up higher on your pubic mound. In either case, the dildo will be fixed against your pubic mound and your clitoris will hang underneath in the cylinder. Proceed carefully as you begin to penetrate your partner. The missionary position works well for this technique, especially if the receptive partner elevates her hips high enough to avoid breaking the cylinder's suction.

Penetration: The Meat of the Matter

There are two basic approaches to penetration with a pumped-up clit: cylinder on and *sans* cylinder. It is difficult to perform penetration once you remove the cylinder, especially if you do not take synthetic testosterone. Difficult yes, but not impossible.

To begin, place a bolo cock ring and a condom around your clit, clitoral hood, and labia minora after you remove the cylinder. Work with your partner to find a position in which your package can be used to its best advantage. The receptive partner on top and the missionary position with the receptive partner propped up on pillows are both good bets. You may not be able to actually insert your genitals into the vagina or anus of your partner, but thrusting may feel quite like penetration nonetheless. Receptive partners who enjoy deep penetration will have to be accommodated in other ways, but both partners can achieve a great deal of genital stimulation from this act alone. If you want to engage in deeper penetration, lubricate your clit and insert it into a dildo that has a small hole in the back of its base, such as Vixen Creations' Treasure Chest; use a harness to hold the dildo against your body.

With the pump cylinder still in place, you can try a hollow latex dildo (such as those made by Doc Johnson) or a cyberskin sleeve. Stuff a bit of cotton or latex into the end of the sleeve and slide it over your cylinder-encased clit. When successful, this method can feel like genital penetration for both partners.

Safety is an important consideration if you want to keep the cylinder on your clit during penetration. *Never insert the cylinder directly into the vagina or anus of your partner, since the metal and hard plastic edges of the cylinder's coupler could cause serious injury.* You can try sheathing your cylinder-encased clit with a vibrator sleeve or a penis extender made from Cyberskin, silicone, or soft plastic. There are a number of toys which can be adapted for this purpose, including the Hot Rod Enhancer and the Senso-Extension made by California Exotic Novelties, and Cyberskin sleeves made by Topco Sales. Fill the end of the hollow tube with fabric or cotton to provide extra cushioning and to take up the slack between the cylinder and the end of the sleeve. Make sure that the sharp edges of the cylinder cannot pierce through the material and scrape your partner's flesh.

Androgens and Long-Term Pumping

Occasional, moderate pumpers need not be concerned about any permanent clitoral growth; after twelve to twenty-four hours, your genitals will return to their normal size. According to the anecdotal experience of long-term, frequent pumpers, however, it is possible to achieve a permanent increase in clitoral size with regular daily use of a hose-pump system, especially when combined with masculinizing hormones (androgens) or over-the-counter testosterone-enhancing products. You should not boost your testosterone levels merely to enjoy the pleasures of pumping, however, for it is simply not necessary. Androgens can have serious consequences for your health, behavior, and appearance, including increased body and facial hair, lowering of the voice, and increased sex drive and aggression. Even if you desire such effects, androgens should only be used under the care of a qualified medical practitioner, as the drugs can cause serious liver and cardiovascular complications.

Anal
Exploits

10

Anal Tension

Dealing with the issue of anal tension is imperative to
great strap-on sex. Just as the muscles in one's neck or
back can become constricted with the day's tension, the
anus can become a repository of the stresses, worries,
and fears that we experience in our day-to-day lives. Yet
this notion can be difficult for many folks to comprehend:
while they may recognize the function of tension in the
muscles of the shoulders, back and neck, they draw a line
between these muscles and those in the anus and genitals, which are just as likely to store this sort of general
tension. Moreover, just as someone may gather an inor-
dinate amount of stress in her neck or jaw, the anus may
be a specific magnet for tension.

Similarly, the anus and rectum are often overly tight due to our attempts to curtail its instinctive urge to release feces when we encounter stress or danger. You see, babies spontaneously defecate when confronted with such threats. As we get older though, we realize that this response is socially inappropriate, and we learn to constrict the muscles of the anus and rectum to prevent this innate function. Thus often as adults, our bodies become an unyielding armor of tensed muscle whenever we feel the urge to defecate. In some folks, this anal tension occurs not only in response to the urge to defecate, but is in effect almost continuously throughout the day. In those of us who have experienced some form of trauma in the anal area—whether from overly strict toilet training or sexual assault—this level of tension may be exacerbated. Dramatically invasive ordeals can leave residual tension which can remain in the body indefinitely if unattended and can severely impede enjoyment of strap-on sex.

What to do? Give heed to the tension level of your anus and external sphincter at different times in the day. Is your anus contracted or relaxed, or somewhere in between? Notice what it feels like when you are faced with stress at work or at home, or as you engage in a relaxing activity, such as taking a hot bath, getting a massage, drinking a glass of wine, or even engaging in warm conversation with a good friend. Does the anus tense up or slacken in response to the way in which your attention is focused? Conversely, when your anal muscles are relaxed, do you feel relaxed emotionally as well? Just as your emotions can influence the level of stress in the body, the body can influence the emotions when conscious attention is paid to it.

The simple exercise described in "Anal Consciousness" below can help get you on the road to anal relaxation.

Even if you're the one doing the strapping, a relaxed rectum will serve to increase the pleasure you experience during strap-on sex.

Anal Consciousness

In his classic book, *Anal Pleasure and Health,* Jack Morin recommends that the following exercise be practiced daily in order to develop a consciousness around the level of anal tension held in your body. Lay on your back and observe your breathing. Then pay attention to your anus. Is it relaxed or contracted? Simply observe it. Now inhale and hold your breath for a few seconds and make your anus as tight as you can; let it relax as you exhale. Imagine blood flooding the area and bringing warmth with it. Repeat if desired.

Anal Hygiene

Many people repress their desire for strap-on anal sex because they fear encountering feces in the bargain. Though there is no foolproof way to avoid that occurrence, there are a number of things you can do to lessen the possibility, as well as to de-escalate any anxiety you may have about it. First off, remember that the rectum is merely a way station for feces which pass through during elimination. In healthy people, there is little if any feces stored in this area. You can use latex gloves and condoms on dildos as a means of lessening any uneasiness you may have about this prospect.

Good anal hygiene requires attention to diet, toilet habits, and cleanliness, as well as the release of tension in the anal area. Your diet should consist of whole grains, fruits, vegetables, and lots of water to insure big, soft, thick, bulky stools. A bit of psyllium husks, either *au naturel* or in a commercial product like Metamucil, can help in this regard as well. Likewise, good toilet habits help ensure both good general health and a clean rectum. When nature calls, don't ignore her missive: get yourself to a bathroom straight away when you feel the urge to go. Also refrain from pushing or straining too hard during elimination. If you frequently feel you must strain your rectum in order to defecate, you are likely holding in your feces too long and/or consuming a diet insufficient in fiber. If you have serious problems in this regard, take steps to resolve them prior to engaging in anal strap-on sex as the receptive partner, since the solid particles in the residual feces may injure your rectal lining when pressed into the surface by the movement of the toy inside you.

Most fecal matter can be removed with a thorough shower or bath. Be certain to cleanse both the outer anal area and the first inch or so inside the anal canal. Wash well with soap and warm water. If further cleaning is desired, a warm water enema or anal douche to clean out your rectum will not hurt you, unless it is contraindicated by your physician. The procedure is simple. First, procure either a douche bulb designed specifically for the purpose of rectal cleansing, or buy a Fleet enema, available at most drugstores. (If you purchase a commercially prepared enema, pour out the contents of the bottle and replace with warm water—the chemicals could irritate the delicate mucous membranes of your rectum.) Then put a bit of water-based lube on the nozzle, carefully insert it into your rectum, and squeeze the warm water into your anal canal and rectum. Hold the water inside your rectum for a few minutes and then release it. You can repeat these steps as needed prior to or after anal strap-on sex. In fact, you may find the process itself to be quite pleasurable.

Anal Penetration

Okay, you're thinking, "My butt is as relaxed as a belly dancer's midriff and as clean as driven snow. When do I get to break out the strap-on?" Well, just hold your horses.

If you're the receptive partner, you may very well want to practice by yourself first with a freestanding toy in order to acquaint yourself with the sensations of anal sex with a dildo. Playing solo is a good way to loosen up, especially for beginners. You can practice relaxing and stimulating your anus without worrying about another person.

Even if you have had anal intercourse with a penis, the sensation is different with an unyielding toy. Says Tim Dunlavy, of Jaguar Books in San Francisco:

> Personally, I have a better orgasm with a dildo than a penis—it makes everything inside me more sensitive. A real dick moves and shapes itself to the ass around it; a dildo does not. A dildo is rigid, and the ass has to arrange itself to accommodate it. I like to use sex with a dildo for foreplay, as it prepares me for my lover's dick. Once he is inside me, I can feel everything way more intensely—if his dick tenses, I can feel it.

When you are ready to have anal strap-on sex, make sure that you are with a partner you can trust, especially if you are the receptive partner. Since the structures of the anus and rectum are rich with nerve endings and the sphincter muscle is often constricted, there is a strong relationship engendered between anal penetration and the thoughts and emotions of the person being penetrated. Consequently, it is especially important that an environment of trust and care be fostered between partners when anal sex will take place, since without that level of care and communication, it is quite possible that real damage will be done.

Flat out, you must never have anal strap-on sex with someone who does not care for your well-being. On the other hand, when that connection *is* in place, the level of trust and caring that accompanies strap-on anal sex is remarkable, and the potential for an interchange of profound emotion is boundless, regardless what the content of that exchange may be.

> When a girl feels as though she trusts me enough to open up her ass to me, it is a wonderful gift of love, innocence, submission.

Setting the Stage

Once you have chosen a partner with whom you feel comfortable, think about when you want anal sex to take place. For instance, you may want to introduce strap-on anal sex in the context of a sex act that you and your partner already enjoy.

> I like to insinuate my interest in his ass way before I'm going to fuck him there—rubbing the opening, resting a finger inside him, or maybe inserting a butt plug in him while I suck his dick.

This method serves two purposes. First, because of the profound relaxation that often accompanies the resolution phase of the sexual arousal cycle—that is, the release of the sexual tension after orgasm—experimenting with anal sex after genital stimulation can be a great idea. Just as the genitals are effected by vasocongestion, the swelling which accompanies sexual excitement and arousal, and myotonia, the process whereby muscle groups collect sexual tension during arousal, so is the anal-rectal area. Sexual activity, in particular orgasm, releases much of that tension and swelling from the structures of the anus and rectum, and thus more readily facilitates anal penetration

Having an orgasm releases muscular tension, and in general makes us both more relaxed and excited at the same time—which is a very good place from which to begin anal penetration.

> After whirling round and round the opening to her ass, I make her feel secure by wrapping my body around hers. I want to make her feel safe, taken care of, appreciated, loved. Before I enter her anus, I rub her breasts as well, and sometimes bring back some of the juice from her pussy to remind her of the intensity and pleasure we just had with sex there.

Second, when you begin your sex session with an activity about which you and your partner feel gratified, you will feel less pressure to push anal sex beyond the bounds of comfort. Since you have already had a sexual "success," neither of you will likely feel as compelled to press the project of anal strap-on sex beyond your physical or emotional limits this particular time out.

Begin your anal play by relaxing the anus through massage and focused breathing. The strapper can massage the outside of the anus, allowing her partner to relax into a sense of trust. Anal massage should be done gently, but firmly. When anal touch is either too harsh or too tentative, it can be difficult for the receptive partner to feel secure with her partner.

Pay plenty of attention to the perineum during anal massage—a great deal of tension can be stored there, which can pose problems during anal penetration. Stroke the perineum gently but firmly from the outside, slowly, not rapidly, in order to relax the area. Often just holding your hand on the perineum can convey a message of trust, peace and relaxation to a partner.

To relax the perineum after initiating penetration with a woman partner, insert a finger into your partner's anus and a finger into her vagina. Slowly and deliberately massge the perineal wall, using both fingers in tandem. With a male receptive partner, insert a finger into the anus and massage his perineal wall by gently pressing against it from inside while supporting the tissue beneath his testicles with your free hand.

During massage, the receptive partner can breathe deeply. Imagine breathing down to your asshole and allowing the breath to open up your anus and rectum. Then bear down to better relax your sphincter muscles and facilitate entry. If you are particularly tense, your partner can hold you in an upright, supported position as you bear down.

Anal Sex in the Digital Age

You will want to begin your anal exploits with the use of your fingers rather than jumping right to the strap-on, especially if you don't have a lot of experience with anal strap-on sex or if your partner is new to you. Rest your finger against your partner's anus as she continues to breathe deeply and to push her anal muscles outward. When you feel her anal muscles relax, you can enter her slowly with one finger. Talk to your partner so that she feels the connection between you; you may even want to breathe with her. Then, on an out breath, enter her very gently but not tentatively, with a well-lubricated finger. As you penetrate her, hold her so that she feels warm and contained. Later, you may want to suck her nipples or apply nipple clamps, add cock rings in the case of a male receptive partner, or combine kissing, biting, genital stroking or vibration—whatever feels good for both of you.

The use of lubricant with anal strap-on sex is imperative: though the rectum does produce a small amount of anal mucous and sweat, it is not enough lubrication to facilitate penetration in most cases. Many people prefer a thick, rich lube, such as Embrace or Maximus, because it adheres to the sides of rectal walls. Don't hesitate to mix two or more water-based lubes if you want to experiment with different densities and textures. In fact, you may want to add a thinner, more slippery lube to the mix, such as ID or Astroglide, as the rate of penetration picks up. Entry and removal are the most challenging aspects of anal penetration. So when you need to add more lube, minimize any discomfort by pulling your fingers out partially, using them as a conduit to conduct the lubricant into your partner's ass, rather than removing them completely.

Once your finger is inserted, move it slowly at first, if at all. You may want to hold it still until your partner becomes accustomed to its presence, especially if she is inexperienced with either anal sex in general or with you as a partner. It is a common sensation for receptive partners new to anal sex to feel the need to defecate with rectal stimulation. Allow your partner to make a trip to the bathroom to reassure herrself. As your partner adjusts to the new stimulation, you will feel the contractions of her relaxation. You can now slowly begin to move your finger back and forth. Continue talking to her—you may even want to describe what you are doing, so that she can feel prepared for each new sensation. Begin moving your fingers more rapidly once you sense that your partner has become relaxed enough to do so.

As the receptive partner, you may prefer to control the action entirely. Try sitting on your partner's finger. Tell him he cannot initiate movement of any kind until you ask him to do so.

You can insert a second finger without completely removing the first, adding more lube in the process. Continue preparing your partner's ass in this way, adding fingers until the anal opening is stretched enough to accept the insertion of the dildo. When you are ready to remove your fingers and insert the toy, be sure to remove them gently. Your partner can help by bearing down as the two of you coordinate the removal of your hand. As with insertion, it is important to remove your fingers slowly but surely.

Gradually increase penetration, stopping or retreating to a more comfortable position if your partner feels pain. Pain is *not* a necessary function of anal sex and ignoring it can lead to damage. The first curve in the rectum is the juncture at which many encounter difficulty. A review of anal anatomy may be helpful. (See Chapter 2, Anatomy). Take care to keep the lines of communication open, stay conscious of the angle of the rectum, and pay heed to *any* pain your partner encounters.

Make sure to avoid short-circuiting your sensations by overindulging in drugs or alcohol. While a glass or two of wine or a toke of pot can release inhibitions and relax muscular tension during anal sex, if you gorge on drugs or drink, your level of sexual response will actually be lessened and most importantly, your response to pain will be numbed. In this state, you can easily cause serious damage to your anal health during anal strap-on sex, since the pain reflex is in place to prevent damage to your anus and rectum.

Strappers may well want to be wearing their strap-on at this point, as you don't want to lose the moment by breaking away to slip into your harness. If you do have to leave to don your rig, don't expect to return to the same level of stimulation you had reached when you left. Instead, go back a few steps and warm up your partner a bit before entering her with your strap-on.

Whether attached to a harness or as a freestanding dildo, you must use toys equipped with a flange for anal sex, since it can be especially difficult to retrieve a toy that slips into the rectum. If a toy does get lodged inside your rectum, don't panic: relax, bear down, and gently push it out with your anal muscles.

Enter the Strap-on

Lube up your dildo! At long last, you're ready for anal strap-on sex. Coat your tool with a good amount of a thick lube that will adhere to the walls of the rectum and to the toy. Then place just the tip of it at the opening to your partner's anus. Let it rest there. This step allows your partner to get accustomed to the idea of being penetrated in the ass by an object larger than a finger and furthers the trust and warmth you have built up while using your hands. Plus, it's just darn sexy. At any rate, continuing the emotional connection of your earlier play in strap-on sex is very important, particularly early on, since your dildo is equipped with neither the warmth or tactility of your hands. Verbal communication can be very important at this point.

Follow the same deep breathing, massage, and muscular contraction techniques discussed above in reference to anal-digital sex. Warm your toy so that your partner's anus will not contract painfully around it. You can soak the dildo in warm water it before you strap it on or rub it vigorously with lube to heat it up with friction. Enter your partner very slowly. After the dildo is in place, hold it still for a moment. Make sure that the angle of the dildo and the angle of your partner's body coincide to avoid poking the curve of her rectum. This is especially important since it is very easy to damage the fragile mucous membrane lining of the rectum. As you move inside your partner, try to visualize the shape and angle of her rectum, which you discovered with your hand.

Once fully inside your partner, hold still again until your partner has indicated either verbally or with his body movements and breathing that he is ready for you to begin to thrust. When you begin to thrust, do so slowly, and speed up only when you sense either by his words or breathing and muscular contractions that he is ready for more intense stimulation.

The receptive partner may well want to take the reigns by sitting astride the dildo; you can ask your partner to wait for your invitation before making any movement.

If you need more lubricant, you needn't pull out completely. Keep at least the tip of the toy inside your partner, and then use the toy as a conduit for the lube. By this point, you may well be ready for something thinner and more slippery to promote more rapid movement. Feel free to experiment with water-based lubes. Remember to keep the lines of communication open, and to adjust your movements or stop them completely if your partner experiences pain. When you are ready to pull out, remove the toy slowly but deliberately. To minimize any discomfort, the receptive partner can breathe deeply and bear down as her partner removes the toy on an out breath.

Toys for Boys

11

Howdy, Sport! If you skipped straight to this chapter in order to glean some information about boys and anal penetration, you just go back to Chapter 1 and start reading! The entire volume is filled with strap-on lore just as relevant to men getting it up the butt as it is to women taking a strap-on in either orifice. This chapter, however, is just for men—straight, bisexual, gay, and transsexual—who would like to wear a strap-on dildo in a harness to penetrate their partners.

Let's begin with the eternal question: Why would a man want to strap it on? Many folks assume that only men with erectile difficulties would want to use a dildo and harness. Balderdash—there are a number of reasons why a man would want to wear a strap-on. He can use a strap-on in conjunction with a hard-on to penetrate more than one partner, or to fill a female partner in both her vagina and her anus, for instance. Of course, instances of "impotence" are a perfect time for a man to slip on his strap-on. But rather than thinking of strap-on use as a way to cope with a medical problem, let's expand our possibilities. You can enjoy using a strap-on whenever you want to be the insertive partner in penetrative sex but don't have an erection. You may have already spent your erection earlier in the evening, your penis may not be in the mood when the rest of you is raring to go, or you may have a clinically diagnosed erectile problem.

Great idea, no? Well sure, but erection issues in general—and strap-on use in particular—can be an intimidating prospect for many men. Why? Well, strap-ons contradict the phallocentrism of Western culture. A lot of men (and their partners) are sure in their heart of hearts that sex is possible *only* with penetration, and penetration is possible *only* with a large, erect penis. This is a heck of a lot of pressure for Peter to live up to. But, let's face it— having an erect dick attached to your hips *can* in fact provide you and your partner with great pleasure, whether the erection is made of flesh or PVC. And with strap-on sex, a man doesn't have to contend with the enormous stress of "performance anxiety." When the focus of sex has shifted from performance to fun and intimacy, anyone who wants to have an erection can have one, any time, any place, and in most any physical condition.

The fact of the matter is that despite the myth of male virility, not all men walk around in a constant state of arousal, prepared to sally forth with an erection on demand just because an opportunity presents itself. There may be times when your partner initiates sex, and though you may want to participate, your penis does not. This is a perfect time to strap-on a dildo or insert your soft dick into a hollow Cyberskin sleeve and give it a go. Or maybe you and your partner want to keep going after you have orgasmed and become soft. Well, you needn't give up the ghost just because your dick needs a rest—keep your rig by the bed and you won't miss a beat. Regardless of the situation, if you and your partner want penetrative sex and your natural equipment is grounded, why not ditch the mythology, take some stress off your dick, and make do with a dildo and harness? You may well become erect once the performance anxiety is alleviated and you have given yourself the permission to enjoy sex nonetheless. This is the happy paradox of strap-on sex for men.

The pressure to produce erections on demand is not the only cause of distress for men and their partners. Oh no, confusing penis size with sexual worth is just as troublesome. Many a man feels chagrined if his penis doesn't extend to porn star proportions. This is unfortunate, especially since porn star dicks—rock hard, semen-spewing, nine and ten inch models—are about as rare among men as size two bodies are among women. And just as photographic images of those waif-like beauties are carefully styled and airbrushed, video images of erect penises are manipulated by lighting and editing to produce penile performances Eros himself would envy. Don't believe the hype. Learn a lesson from experienced female strappers who, on the whole, have much less emotional investment in the dimensions of their package: the size dildo receptive partners prefer varies enormously based on physiology and desire, and by no means is bigger always better.

In other words, the degree to which your penis size will effect your partner's pleasure is pure happenstance—some female and male receptive partners, for reasons of physiology, love to be filled to the brim with something thick and long. But just as many prefer those a phallus, whether organic or synthetic, that is thinner and shorter. Many folks enjoy a range of sizes which they can accom-

Gay Boys and Their Toys

Here's the expert advice of the boys at Jaguar Bookstore in San Francisco: Tim Dunlavy, Sergio Pineda, Toby and Tristan Paris (who, by the way, is the famous boy bottom, starring in Mercury Rising *and* The Big Thrill.*) If anyone has their fingers on the pulse of gay dildo aficionados, it's these gentlemen:*

- TRISTAN: "Some men are bottoms with penetration, wanting only to be penetrated, and others are tops, wanting only to penetrate their partners. Many, though, are versatile."

- TOBY: "Some gay men just really love toys. They want to enhance their sex life and try something new or different, since dildos come in a lot of sizes, textures and colors. Some may buy a dildo because his boyfriend is out of town and he wants to use it to masturbate. Suction cups fitted on the bottom of the dildos are great for solo sex play. You can stick them to the floor or the wall." Tristan agrees: "If I don't want to go out, spend money, or buy drinks, I can use my friend at home."

- TIM: "Some gay men have taboos about dildo use, just like any segment of the population. They think that dildos are dirty, kinky, or naughty." (Perhaps these prohibitions can serve to make their use more exciting for other gay men!)

- TIM: "Most customers are size queens. When you are buying your first dildo, you will likely want to steer away from big dildos. An 8-inch dildo is not the same as an 8-inch penis. They don't bend or move like real dicks—you have to bend and move to accommodate them."

- TRISTAN: "If I want something large and I am with a guy with a small dick, I bring my toys, so I am always happy. I may warm up with my partner's dick and then use my toys, or I may ask him to perform double penetration with his dick and a dildo at the same time. I want to make sure he feels comfortable with the toys I bring along."

- Some gay men use dildos with a partner for reasons of safer sex. Anal-penile intercourse is an extremely efficient way for the HIV virus to be transmitted, and even though much of the risk is eliminated through the conscientious use of condoms, many men still prefer to use dildos.
- Tim remarks that sometimes gay men use dildos as a warm up for penile-anal sex, or after their partner has ejaculated and gone soft. In fact, many bottoms remark in fact that anal sex is more pleasurable after they themselves have come.
- Sergio is often with men who only want to bottom during anal play. Just in case he is with such a partner and he wants to be penetrated, he "makes sure he always brings his dildos along."
- Tristan says that many gay men like to use double-headed dildos, especially if they both want to bottom. "During three-ways, the bottoms can get on all fours butt-to-butt, and the top can use the toy on them both at the same time."
- Though much of dildo use among gay men is with freestanding toys, just like straight men, some gay and bi men use strap-ons after their initial erection is spent, because of erectile difficulties, because they are not in the mood for penile intercourse with their partner, or because they want to penetrate more than one partner at a time.
- Tim adds that allowing a partner to penetrate you anally has special significance for many men in the gay community. "To open yourself anally to a man's penis may symbolize a great opening of the heart as well." Some men may desire to have the stimulation of anal penetration without engaging in this sort of emotional vulnerability, and thus choose to use a dildo instead.
- Some gay men prefer dildos to penises when it comes to anal penetration. Tristan says: "I don't always come when I am being fucked by a man's dick, but I always do with a dildo."

modate and enjoy. Some receptive partners go for variety—perhaps needing something larger or smaller at different times in their sexual lives, a particular relationship, or even a particular day. And certainly many women prefer a different sized rod for anal rather than vaginal penetration. While your standard equipment comes in one size, dildos come in just about any size or proportion from something resembling a pinkie to something resembling a forearm. Thus strap-ons (and freestanding dildos) can be of enormous value when you want to diversify your penile portfolio.

Okay, now that we've got some of the reasoning squared away, let's move onto more practical issues: how does one strap a dildo and harness rig over male genitals? Which style harness is the best choice? Well, the most likely contender is the jockstrap-style harness. With this model, your genitals can hang between the straps rather than be constricted by a strap dividing them to either side. The front plate of the harness holds the dildo onto the hard surface of your pubic mound, and the straps wrap around your thighs rather than between your legs, allowing your nature-made parts to swing freely.

Some men prefer a thong-style harness because they actually enjoy the sensation of the center strap holding the penis and testicles taut to one side. An added advantage with this style harness is that you can attach a cuff to the center strap to hold a butt plug inside your ass while strapping. You can also use the O-ring as a cock ring when the dildo is not in use.

Thigh harnesses are a good choice if you would rather not contend with the issue of fitting your genitals into any particular configuration whatsoever. They also allow you to penetrate two or more partners at the same time, situating one receptive partner on each knee, for instance.

If you want to use a rig to penetrate your female partner in her anus and vagina at the same time, you will
have to arrange your erection and an erect dildo in very
close quarters. The majority of fellows who try this trick
use a jockstrap style harness. With this harness, the straps
go around the your erection and situate the dildo on your
pubic mound directly above and parallel to your penis.
You can decide whether you want your penis to be inside
your partner's vagina and the dildo inside her ass, or vice
versa depending on the position you choose. For example, in the missionary position, your penis will be inside
her ass and the dildo inside her vagina. In the rear entry
position, this order will be reversed. Naturally, you can
take size preferences into account when deciding what
should go where.

Regardless of which model you choose, and how you
want to play, consider trying a strap-on and having yourself a hoe-down!

Strap-On Sex and Your Sexual Imagination

12

Hitherto, dear reader, we have addressed the basic apparatii, both human and synthetic, with which you should be conversant to make the most of your strap-on sex experience. We have considered the mechanics of the prospect: angle, staying power and positions, as well as a few auxiliary endeavors such as packing, strapper stimulation, and clit pumping. Yet the whole of strap-on sex consists of far more than a consideration of either the raw materials which power it—or the merits of choosing side-by-side over doggy style. One of the most important, and certainly one of the most interesting components of strap-on play is the sexual imagination you bring to the enterprise. To wit: the process involved in moving from your inner notions about strap-on sex—your passions, fears, emotions, desires, and fantasies—to a place of making it real, and really gratifying for you and your partner.

How can you transform your feelings about strap-on sex—your passions, fears, desires, and fantasies—into a gratifying reality for yourself and your partner? This chapter will help you to explore your libido and infuse your strap-on play with the passion you uncover there.

You may be thinking that you just want use a strap-on to penetrate your partner with your hands free and have full-body contact while you do it. And that is a fine ambition. Convenience is certainly enhanced by strap-on sex. Yet even if your attraction to strap-on sex is based on utility, the endeavor can be enhanced if you connect your fantasies and emotions to the physical experiences of your body. If you're wearing the dildo and harness, you might want to explore the idea of getting in touch with your "inner dick." When you are aware of your inner dick, you can develop greater finesse and skill as an insertive partner because you will become more in tune with the length, breadth, and texture of the dildo. The more familiar you are with both the reality and the fantasy of that organ, the more your strap-on will become a conduit for exchanging energy and sensuality between you and your partner—and less an inert device. Strengthening the relationship between your sexual imagination and your tactile arousal can help you experience a stronger connection with your partner and greater physical pleasure from strap-on sex.

I would say that visual and aural stimulation are what bring me closest to my inner dick. When she is writhing and wet and waiting for me to fill her hungry hole, my inner dick is with me. When she whispers urgently, "fuck me," my inner dick takes over and transforms my body into a hot throbbing cock.

Foster Your Sexual Imagination

A dildo itself is an inanimate object; it comes to life only when you imbue it with the force of your passion and that of your partner. The actual toy serves as a divining rod for the feelings you have about your sexuality in general and penetration in particular. It is a physical metaphor for your unique inner sexuality. It may reflect normative cultural assumptions, such as the notion that the phallus represent masculinity or even dominance, or it may convey something else entirely. Perhaps you are a feminine dominant woman, and your phallus conveys your sexual power without overtones of masculinity. Or maybe you are a gay female-to-male transsexual with fantasies of submission, and your phallus represents your masculinity without overtones of dominance. Maybe your inner dick has little to do with gender or power, but serves as a Tantric conduit for transmitting energy between yourself and your partner. A dildo is just a piece of material, much like a penis is just a piece of flesh; its significance is enlarged by your imagination.

Different people connect to their inner sexuality in different ways. Ask yourself what settings and mechanisms will help you bring forth your sexual inner life in the context of strap-on sex. Will you feel most comfortable making sexual discoveries when you are alone or with a particular partner? It is up to you whether you want to take time alone to find your inner dick or whether you want to enlist the help of your mate.

You may be most comfortable shopping for sex toys with a platonic friend rather than with a lover. You may prefer to conduct your explorations alone. Touching yourself in ways you find sexually gratifying and paying conscious attention to the images that pass through your consciousness may help bring your most deeply buried sexual feelings to the surface. In addition, being away from your partner for this kind of investigation can give you the opportunity to approach her later with a sexy new surprise.

Alternatively, you may have greater access to your inner sexuality if your partner joins you in selecting a strap-on or attending an instructional workshop. Many people can best get in touch with their sexual imagination through partnered sex. Listening to your partner's fantasies or playing lovers' games such as *Passion Play* or Laura Corn's *101 Quickies* can also be a great way to tap into your libidinous mind. Step back for a moment and think about which approach would feel best to you—perhaps it is a combination of both. If you do decide to bring your partner along for the ride, make sure you feel confident that she will offer loving support as you go through the process.

Either way, solo or with a lover, you may find your inspiration in written erotica. From Sappho's tributes to her beloved and to *Lady Chatterly's Lover* to this month's issue of *Penthouse Forum*, erotica has always existed. And why not? Sex can be one of life's greatest ecstasies—it's no surprise that so many writers want to share their sexual discoveries and that so many readers devour these contributions as fodder for their own sexual epiphanies. Whether at your local independent bookstore, a sex specialty store, or through an online bookseller, you can find scads of smut to get your home fires burning. Or perhaps you are inspired by love stories that are more romantic and less explicitly sexual. If so, you're certainly not alone—many folks find it easier to identify with the erotic sensibilities of the characters in less graphic material.

If sexy short stories are not your thing, you may prefer audio erotica, uttered by a breathy starlet or some bass-voiced hunk, your own journals, or even nonfiction essays about sex. Look for books about sexual practices that fascinate you, such as Tantra, oral sex, or polyamory.

There is no end to the selection of visual material available to stir up your sexual imagination. Sexually-oriented videos and DVDs number in the tens of thousands. They range from standard mainstream porn to feminist heterosexual videos to slick gay boy-on-boy flicks to low-budget films made by and for lesbians. You can find how-to films on everything from masturbation to bondage.

The World Wide Web offers a wealth of inspiration for getting in touch with your inner dick or quintessential orifice. The Web has rapidly become an extraordinary resource for sexual material of all sorts; simply type your favorite sexual subjects into a search engine, and you will likely get more responses than you'll know what to do with. If you prefer your erotic stimuli in a non-digital medium, sexual artwork such as erotic painting, sculpture, or photography can provide you with plenty of fodder for your imagination. And don't forget the old standbys, pornographic magazines. Even a trip to a sex toy store to absorb the atmosphere can increase your awareness of your inner sexuality.

Likewise, attending strip clubs or sex parties—whether alone, with a partner, or with platonic friends—or venturing out on the town to cruise for an appealing stranger can take you places you've never been before.

Some people prefer the contemplative approach, using meditation to conjure up their inner sexual fantasies. Taking a vacation by yourself or with a partner—whether in a sumptuous big city hotel or a Motel 6 half an hour down the highway—can liberate your sexual imagination from the confines of your daily routine. Indeed, being away from the habits of home can often make your most meaningful erotic ideas stand out in sharp relief.

A counselor, sex therapist, or sex educator—or dominatrix, if that is more your style—can help you make a significant shift in your inner sexual life. Often the input of a third party in a professional setting can enable you to make dramatic breakthroughs in how you approach your own sexuality.

So you've found a porn movie or Victorian novella that strikes your fancy, or trekked to a contemplative mountain retreat—or the nearest sleazy motel. What do you do with the strap-on sex fantasy you have discovered in your forays?

Perhaps, as a female, you have discovered a fantasy in which you are a man fucking your girlfriend with your own dick. As a biological male, you might see yourself as a two-dicked creature able to fill both your girlfriend's vagina and ass. Perhaps you have a fantasy of penetrating your boyfriend in a new way. Maybe you are a married woman and envision yourself being fucked by a male stranger at a truck stop. Or perhaps you are a sexually dominant butch dyke and imagine yourself being taken by your femme wife, her brother, or both.

What do you do if your fantasies are illegal, or are in conflict with your political identity, the boundaries established by your current relationship, or your personal sense of ethics? Perhaps themes of violence or incest come up in your fantasies. If you are an experienced S/M player, maybe your reveries are surprisingly vanilla. Possibly your gender or sexual orientation is considerably different in your imagination than in everyday life. Maybe your fantasies involve people other than your partner, or exclude your partner altogether by virtue of his or her anatomy. Or perhaps the images that you find most exciting stand in direct contrast to the role you usually play in your sexual relationships. Your sexual fantasies may fill you with delight and anticipation, but when they raise conflicts between your desires and the life you have chosen, they may also fill you with consternation.

Sexual fantasies are funny things. Sometimes they are

quite literal—you fantasize about penetrating your boyfriend's ass because you want to penetrate his ass, and you feel little ambiguity about that fact. But at other times, sexual fantasies can take on a highly symbolic function and stand in for other elements in your subconscious. These fancies may be comprised of various images and yearnings that have made their way onto the theatrical stage of your conscious thought. They may be influenced by early childhood experiences, sex with past lovers, erotic books and videos, the sight of a sexy coworker, cultural and subcultural taboos, or the media, or they may be chiefly a product of your own sexual imagination.

> My favorite fantasy is of me wearing a dildo and harness while fully clothed, and having a man on his knees sucking on it while I stand watching him. Why? It is so hot to see his vulnerability and feel the power of being sucked. It is so erotic and awesome.

Some of these fantasies fall squarely within the realm of your actual experience, as when you replay a greatest hits reel of sex with a particular partner. Others would horrify you if they actually came true, such as fantasies of rape, castration, or radical gender transformation. These images can be bewildering if they place you in a situation or with partners very different from those in your day-to-day life. For example, you may be a feminine woman with occasional daydreams of being a man getting a blow job from a leatherboy in an alley. Or perhaps you are a burly dominant man in your everyday life, but are thrilled by the fantasy of yourself as a woman bent over the nearest piece of furniture and getting fucked for all you're worth. Maybe your fantasies defy the laws of physics and human physiology altogether—you see yourself as an animal or a creature from a sci-fi flick with sex organs not currently represented on this planet.

I am a bisexual boy and I had a dream about a lesbian friend. She was wearing jeans and a tank top (very butch) and I was dressed like a cheerleader, but was still a boy. I jumped her and unzipped her jeans to find a huge cock. She was on her back and I mounted her and got fucked wonderfully hard until I came all over her chest. It was a hot dream. I never told her about it.

If are you the one accustomed to doing the penetrating, you may be alarmed by your desire to be penetrated. Perhaps you fear you are too vulnerable in that position, or that you will no longer feel sufficiently dominant, masculine, or both. Maybe you are concerned that your partner will consider you less than adequate if she knows the content of your fantasies. Perhaps you are female and imagine yourself having a dick with which to penetrate your partner. Do you worry that this means that you are something other than female or feminine? Perhaps receptiveness is conflated with femininity or penetration is tied to masculinity in your conception of your identity or your relationship. Or maybe fantasies involving persons of the "wrong" gender raise concerns about your sexual orientation. How can you realize your newly discovered desires without threatening the stability of either your sexual identity or your existing relationships?

I am a butch dyke, and that means that my cock is of my experience and not of flesh and blood. When I am strapped and packing, there is one part of me that is acutely aware that my cock is a hunk of silicone, held in place with leather or nylon—that it is not truly, literally, objectively a part of me...yet at the same time it is absolutely me.

Conflicts that arise from your sexual fantasies can feel very threatening indeed. It is natural to conclude that fantasies that are in direct opposition to your sexual reality will profoundly disrupt and destabilize your sexual orientation and relationships, or that they must quickly be repressed and sent back into the subconscious abyss from which they originated. However, this need not be the case. It is certainly possible that deep exploration into your sexual consciousness may lead you toward dramatic changes in your current relationship or even in your sexual orientation or gender identity. If this movement brings you closer to a sense of authenticity, it definitely bears further investigation. Often though, such drastic measures are not necessary. Even if the specific details of your sexual fantasies cannot be actualized—because they are illegal, unethical, outside the parameters of your relationships or identity, or simply physically impossible—sometimes the essence of these visions can still be realized through responsible, consensual sexual activity that falls within the limits of the agreements you have made with yourself and your partners.

Safe, Sane and Consensual

You can shape your fantasies into a format that works for you, and that is in accord with your lifestyle, your partner situation, your sexual and gender identity, the legal system, your ethics and values, and your real physiology, and the laws of gravity. You may be able to realize the essence underlying your fantasies, even if you cannot actualize specific details. You may wonder, for example, how you can reconcile your fantasies of being penetrated by a man with your commitment to your monogamous relationship with a woman. Or perhaps you are concerned about recurring inappropriate fantasies such as sex with young people, rape, or coercing sex from an employee. Many folks have taboo sexual fantasies such as these.

Consider taking a page from S/M subcultures. Sadomasochism? Yes, indeed. S/M practitioners have much to teach us about bringing sexual fantasies to life in safe and fulfilling ways. Depending on your experience, it may seem frightening to apply the tenets of S/M to your sexual activity, but there are many excellent general S/M principles that have nothing to do with pain or bondage. A cardinal rule of S/M is that fantasies should be brought to life in a safe, sane, and consensual manner. For example, because young children cannot provide meaningful, informed consent, it is not acceptable for adults to engage in sexual activity with children. However, if your fantasies include themes such as vast age differences, corporal punishment, or parental nurturing, it is possible to find a willing adult partner to help you transfer the essence of your fantasies into a legally and ethically acceptable form. While raping or abusing one's partner is clearly reprehensible, the same physical acts done as part of a negotiated, consensual, controlled scenario is a different thing entirely. A basic understanding of S/M principles can help you to think of sex as a theatrical construct in which you and your partner can safely and sanely allow your sexual fantasies to fuel your activities. You may find that the fulfillment of your sexual desires is not only an end in itself, but also a means of connecting more deeply with your partner. When your partner not only accepts, but relishes your fantasies, you can experience new levels of fun, passion, and intimacy in your relationship.

Nothing pleases me more than sucking my Daddy off, so I'd have to say my favorite scene is when I am on my knees so I can use my mouth on her cock. My second favorite position is on my hands and knees, so Daddy can fuck my pussy or my ass.

Gender Transformation

Themes of gender transformation are a common element of strap-on play. If in fact you want to change your sex in your day-to-day life, you will likely experience consistent, deep-seated desires for sex reassignment. However, most people who have genderbending fantasies do not wish to permanently alter their sex. Instead, their reveries more likely indicate a wish to occupy some metaphorical position of dominance or submission, masculinity or femininity, or multigendered or nongendered space that is not a part of their current day-to-day reality.

> I think what turns me on about blow jobs is the fact that it's transgressive—a woman isn't supposed to do that to another woman, a woman isn't supposed to want that from another woman. It's supposed to be one of those things in the realm of male privilege, that which goes with having a fixed, relatively irremovable dick. It feels really right to me to give that privilege, the gift of a blow job, to another woman. It's a way for me to give my partner this precious gift of my feminine body, actions, and response. Not because I want her to be a man, but because society says there's a lot of things we as people born in female bodies aren't supposed to have. I say fuck that— a blow job is my gift to give.

Consider the case of a man who is in a monogamous relationship with a woman, yet while masturbating envisions being anally penetrated by a penis. Does this mean that he is really gay, or at least bisexual? How can he fulfill his fantasies while staying within the parameters he and his partner have established for their relationship? What is he really seeking? How can he create the experience he desires with his partner? Maybe he feels he bears an unfair share of the sexual responsibility in his relationship. Perhaps he is in a position of authority during the workday and relishes the idea of giving up power to his mate at night Or maybe he just desires the stimulation of anal penetration, and the only cultural archetype on which his imagination can focus is a penis. If his partner is so inclined, the use of a dildo and harness could create an exciting opportunity to utilize the power of his fantasies to energize their relationship. In fact, she may harbor her own fantasies that complement those her partner has shared.

Finding Your Inner Dick (Or Quintessential Orifice)

After you have plumbed your sexual imagination and devised a way to make your fantasies work for you and your partner, the next task is to transform your strap-on fantasies into real bodily experiences. Purchase a dildo and harness, if you don't already have one. Select a dildo that will be comfortable and appealing to both you and your partner. Give yourself time to try it on and see how it coincides with your vision of your inner dick. Be sure to stock up on lubricant and latex. (If there is no suitable sex toy store where you live, you can order products using the Web. If you go this route, make sure to do some research in advance since you won't be able to handle or try on products before you buy them. See the Resources.)

Strap on your dildo and harness. Grab your favorite sex toys, erotica, or whatever gets you off. Exploration of your sexual anatomy can help you visualize a connection between your sexual imagination and the package you have riding on your pubic mound. As you feel yourself becoming aroused, pay careful attention to the sensations in your body. Note the feeling of fullness in your pelvis as it swells with blood and other fluids. Register the sensation of your clitoris and crura or penis as it becomes erect, as well as the position and contractions of your PC muscles. Some people experience sexual arousal as a rising sensation in their genital area, and this perception can be particularly conducive to experiencing the inner dick. Put on your harness and dildo and check yourself out in a mirror. Add some clothes that make you feel sexy. You may well feel a bit silly at first, but that awkward feeling is a function of sexual novelty and will likely dissipate as you become more sexually aroused and gain more experience. Continue to stimulate your body while wearing the rig. If you plan to use gadgets designed for strapper stimulation, go ahead and try them out. Put some lubricant on your hands and stroke the dildo as though it were a penis, and touch your body beneath the harness. Visualize a morphing of your clitoral structure or your pubic mound as it extends into the dildo, making it your own.

If you are seeking to be penetrated by a partner wearing a strap-on dildo, you can also benefit by exploring the connection between your sexual anatomy and the sex toy strapped to your partner's body. Feel free to use erotica or whatever else helps arouse you. You may wish to wear clothes that make you feel sexy. Stroke around the entrance to the orifice of your choosing to bring blood and other fluids to the area. Select the dildo you want to use; try strapping it onto a pillow or some other surface to facilitate this solo exercise. Break out the lubricant and mount the dildo. Experiment with different positions and determine what works well for you. The information you obtain will be invaluable during strap-on sex with a partner. Once you reach a sexual rhythm, visualize the desires and fantasies you uncovered earlier and integrate them with the physical pleasure you are feeling—it is in this nexus that your "quintessential orifice" can be found.

Dear Fairy Butch,

Whoa, what's the deal with all of these sex toys I read about in dyke erotica? At first I was turned off by the idea, but the more that I think about it, the more I want to check them out. There's a lesbian-owned store in the city I live in, and I really want to visit, but I am intimidated. Any tips?

—Sequestered in Seattle

Dear Sequestered:

Well, bully for you, Cupcake—sex toys can provide you with more fun than a barrel of monkeys drunk on moonshine! If you live in the vicinity of a customer-oriented toy store (see the Resources), it's worth a bit of anxiety-quelling to get your tush through their doors. These folks pride themselves on providing superb customer service, products of the highest quality, and a light, educational atmosphere amenable to your comfort.

A few pointers:

1. Shop only when you are in an relaxed and happy mood; tension tends to perpetuate itself.

2. Remember, other customers are there for the same reasons as are you, and the store staff has seen it all.

3. Determine whether you would be more comfortable there with a lover or friend, or if you would prefer to fly solo.

4. Go during a slow time in the retail week; early in the day on Mondays and Tuesdays is usually a good bet.

5. Promise yourself that your first trip will be a short one, say 20 minutes, and make plans to reward your bravery afterward.

Then breathe deeply, circle the block three times, and make your way down the road to sex toy ownership, Sugar!

XOXOXOXO,

Fairy Butch

Bringing It Home: Communicating With Your Partner

13

By now you have scoured the recesses of your psyche and have divined the nature of your desires around strap-on sex. Perhaps you harbor a vision of penetrating your husband with your fantasy dick, or maybe you simply have a yen for the no-hands convenience of strap-on sex. Possibly you are enamored of the idea of your wife taking you from behind with her strap-on, or have thought about your girlfriend laying beneath you, inviting you to engulf her erect dildo. Whether you fancy yourself as the pitcher or the catcher, the next step is to share your desires with your partner. Though it can be challenging to navigate the sometimes rocky terrain of sexual communication, especially when communicating ideas that are new, unusual, or taboo, many folks find that they refine their sexual desires in the process, and are brought closer to their partners for the effort. You may in fact be pleasantly surprised to find that your mate's desires complement your own, or even expand on the strap-on themes you had in mind.

Communication Roadblocks

Let's begin at the beginning, with our ideas about sex and the models for sexual communication that we develop as children. Stereotypes and cautionary tales you have absorbed from your parents, schools, the media, religion, and childhood peers can dramatically limit the possibilities for sexual fulfillment. The seeds planted in the fertile soil of our youthful curiosity can have profound consequences for our ability to communicate about sex as adults. In fact, many of us bring to adulthood a notion of sexual communication characterized by using our child's imagination to fill in the gaps of adult conversation, peeks at porno mags and *Baywatch*, and tell-all recess sessions delivered by elementary school playground experts. Many of us receive little honest, effective information about sex as children, and much of what we are offered focuses on the potential perils of sexuality, such as disease and unwanted pregnancy. Although it is important to consider the hazards associated with sexual contact, limiting our sexual communication solely to the realm of risk management does little to enhance sexual pleasure.

Many people have been socialized to believe that communicating their sexual desires to their partner is brazen, demanding, or unsexy. The assumption behind these notions is that by adulthood we should have gained sufficient sexual insight to intuitively make our partner's sexual fantasies come true. Few among us enjoyed this experience of adolescence. Yet sexual technique—like any other skill—is learned, and sexual communication is an integral part of our education. Don't misunderstand me, your instincts can lead you to profound places in your sexuality. But sexual communication with our partners, along with directed self-exploration, workshops, and instructional books and videos, can refine our natural instincts, allowing us to achieve a much greater level of sexual satisfaction.

You may fear that you will hurt or offend your partner by conveying your sexual desires. Perhaps you are afraid that your partner will reject you if she knows the content of your sexual fantasies. Or maybe you are worried that that he will be made uncomfortable or feel excluded by your secret sexual dreams. Perhaps you are concerned that she will be insulted if you suggest new ways of being sexual, as if by doing so you are revealing that you were unhappy with the sex you shared up to this point. This can be tricky territory, particularly if you have not already established effective sexual communication habits. Well, there are a variety of approaches you might try, whether your partner is yours for the night or for life.

Turn the Beat Around

How can you break through the many barriers to sexual communication and lovingly and effectively convey your desires for strap-on play to your partner? There is no single method that works for everyone; there are many unique styles of sexual communication, each of which works well for some people and in some situations. Contrary to popular belief, outright explication is not the only means through which you can express your sexual needs, nor suss out the needs of your partner, though it is highly effective for many people. The best method for you and your partner is the one that makes you feel most understood by your partner and that allows you to best understand his or her sexual needs and desires as well. While some folks find it effective to talk explicitly with their partners about the things that turn them on and the new sexual practices they would like to try, others have developed indirect or nonverbal communication tactics to get their point across.

> Strap-ons are easy. When I want to get fucked, I just say, "Honey, go put your dick on." When she wants a bigger dick she says, "Can we use that one instead?"

> I'm standing with my back to my girlfriend, and the harness straps are laced between my buttocks. She and I both know that something dangerous and decadent awaits.

Some folks brainstorm with their partners about new things they would like to try. Others like to write down their fondest fantasies, whisper them in their partner's ear during sex, or share them over a candlelit dinner. Still others prefer to work in an element of surprise by bringing home a new strap-on toy or hiding sexy notes in their partner's coat pocket.

> I sometimes introduce the idea of strap-on sex to a partner by "accidentally" letting a dildo fall out of my bag during dinner.

Some relish the permission granted by lovers' games, such as *Enchanting Evening*, or Laura Corn's *101 Nights of Great Sex*, which can help people learn more about their sexual proclivities and those of their partner. Many people like to talk about their sexual desires with a third party such as a friend, a counselor, or members of a support group to flesh out the content of their desires prior to approaching their partner with a sexual proposal. Some initiate the discussion by engaging their mates in a conversation about sexual activities of others, whether in the news or in the apartment next door.

Sex Bundles

Each of us starts out with a tacit sexual communication package associated with the gender identity or sexual orientation we present to our partners. Simply by identifying as a member of a particular group—such as Midwestern straight guys or bisexual college women—we communicate a set of sexual standards and assumptions. If you are a very butch-looking lesbian, there is already an established cultural precedent for donning a strap-on dildo. But if you are a heterosexual suburban housewife, your model for strap-on use is probably less clear.

Yet note this vital caveat: You have the freedom to mold cultural archetypes to specifically reflect your own individual identity, either playing up certain aspects which work for you or rejecting established sexual and gender stereotypes. Common cultural models represent only a small segment of the possible ways of being sexual as a heterosexual woman, a gay leatherman, or a member of a monogamous couple. Some of these paradigms are deeply entrenched in our culture, such as the fallacious notion that in all heterosexual couplings the man always does the penetrating and only the woman is penetrated. By rejecting certain elements typically associated with your particular gender package, and mixing in new spices not usually found there, you can create new ways of being sexual that reflect your unique identity. A femme dyke with a raging hard-on? You bet! A straight man who loves to get plugged in the ass doggy style? Why not? As long as you act with respect toward yourself and your partner, the parameters of your sexual repertoire need only be limited only by your imagination and desires.

Effective Communication Models

Okay, enough of the philosophy and the pep talk, how about some hardcore tips? There are two basic aspects to consider when it comes to communicating about strap-on sex: initiating the topic, and deepening your connection with your partner during the act itself. Below are several ideas for improving sexual communication. You may find that by combining elements of various methods or creating entirely new adaptations, you will discover a unique communication style that best suits your needs and inclinations.

Bringing Up the Topic

THE WRITER'S WAY:

The literary approach is perfect for those who enjoy the written word. Write down some encouragement regarding strap-on sex. This can be as simple as a sexy reminder note in your wife's briefcase or as elaborate as a scripted fantasy scenario. If your partner finds your suggestion intriguing, you can work strap-on sex into next sexual encounter. Use lyrical writing if it suits you, or get down and dirty if that's more your style. Try penning your fantasy scenario on a piece of parchment, sending it through the mail, or reading it aloud to your mate in front of the fireplace

YES, NO, AND MAYBE LISTS:

This common S/M technique can be a great icebreaker for people of any sexual persuasion. Draw a grid on a piece of paper with three columns labeled "yes," "no," and "maybe." Write down whatever sexual activities you can think of—including, of course, strap-on sex—and mark which of the three columns they fall into for you. Make a sheet for yourself and one for your partner.

Dear Fairy Butch,

I am a fledgling 22-year-old bottom and I have just had a wonderful experience with the femme fatale dom of my dreams! She evidently enjoyed my company as well because she responded favorably to my request for a second date. Needless to say, I am elated. However, this situation does pose an etiquette dilemma for me. Since she took complete control in our first encounter, I don't know who should plan this next scene: her, because she's the top, or me, since I initiated the date. I'm pretty new to the top/bottom thing and I'm not sure how to proceed in these matters. It really turns me on to do her bidding, and I really want to please her. I would be ever so indebted for your help in this affair.

—Nervous Baby Bottom

Dear Nervous:

Congratulations! That this fabulous creature invited you back to play should serve to quell some of the anxieties that are furrowing your brow. If you would like to plan the scene, call her, or better yet, send a polite, well-penned note asking if she would honor you with her presence at a particular place and time. If she reserves the privilege of determining these details, then you'll know that she expects to retain complete control for now.

If she does deign to consent, then prepare the scene to perfection: make your play space enticing and fill it with implements that strike your fancy. You might want to have tasty foods on hand, and you should certainly have the necessary safer sex materials and lubricant at the ready. Tops vary in both their preferences and expectations. It is quite possible that she'll find the relief from such ministrations to be a refreshing and charming change of pace.

XOXOXOXO,

Fairy Butch

Decide whether you will each fill out your list privately or whether you would prefer to do so together. This technique can be an excellent catalyst for initiating a discussion about strap-on sex and other new things you'd like to try.

LOVERS' GAMES:
Sexy board games can be great fun and a great way to broach new topics far beyond your typical sexual discourse. A good place to start might be with Good Vibration's Love Checks, an inexpensive set of vouchers bearing various sexual requests and favors to be exchanged between partners, such as "This certificate entitles the bearer to one hour of receiving whatever sexual stimulation he desires." Arrange the game so that you get the opportunity to divulge your strap-on fantasy; don't worry about stacking the deck—all's fair in love and war.

You can make up your own game in which each partner gets to plan a sexual evening complete with her choice of location, acts, and implements. Use your partner's "yes," "no," and "maybe" list to help you. You may want to play out a particular fictional or historical scenario or adopt a character whose experience is very different from your own. Setting a time limit in advance can give you the freedom to really let loose, since you know the action will have a definite beginning and ending. In any case, the novelty of sex as perceived through such fictional devices can add an exciting new flavor to the encounter.

My girlfriend named her dildo Charming so that she could work it into polite conversation without others knowing.

THIRD-PARTY PROJECTION:
Third-party projection involves using the experience of other people to initiate a conversation about strap-on sex

with your partner. For example, bring up the Ricki Lake show segment you saw (or wish you saw) yesterday featuring sex toy sellers, or mention that you stumbled across an article in *Playboy* that stated that prostate stimulation has been scientifically proven to improve a man's urogenital health. Once the topic is on the table, tie it into a discussion about your own sexual relationship by asking your partner what he or she thinks about strap-on sex. Or ask your partner about his most fantastic sexual dream, then offer your strap-on sex scenario for his consideration. You might be thrilled to discover some commonalties between your partner's fantasies and your own; or at the very least glean a few revelations for future use.

THE SEX TOY SHOPPING EXPEDITION:
Going to a sex toy store with your partner can be an excellent way to bring up the topic of strap-on sex. If you are lucky enough to live in a city with a customer-oriented, new-generation toy store, you have an excellent opportunity to express your interest in dildos and harnesses. If you are too shy to bring up the subject of sex toy shopping with your partner, tell her you would like her help in picking out a gift for a friend. While there, meander over to the strap-on section and see if the toys spark your partner's interest. Ask her if she has ever considered using a dildo and harness. If you feel too uncomfortable bringing up the subject in public, initiate the conversation later in the day. If you don't live near a comfortable sex toy store, obtain a mail-order catalog from Good Vibrations, Toys in Babeland, or Xandria, and make sure your partner sees you perusing it.

> *My first strap-on experience was with a man. We had been experimenting with anal play and role reversal. I was working at a sex shop at the time,*

and had lots of access to all sorts of toys. We picked out a long, thin red dildo and a purple harness. Fucking him was one of the most intense experiences I had ever had. I felt powerful.

SEXUAL EDUCATION RESOURCES:
The presence of a sexual education book—such as this one—on your coffee table will surely spark some comment from your partner about strap-on sex. If this scheme is too contrived for your tastes, try wrapping the book as a gift for your partner or bringing it out for show-and-tell at an appropriate time. Although a book will send your partner an unambivalent message, it will likely be less threatening than a full strap-on ensemble. Alternatively, bring home *Bend Over Boyfriend*, or another video which showcases strap-on sex. If you happen to have picked up a strap-on sex rig in addition to your video purchase, you might want to reveal it to him at this time.

I love using porn to communicate what I want from my lover. I choose something that I know will feature plenty of the kind of action I want to have with my boyfriend, and then just let the sex on the screen help get us moving in the same direction.

THE PACK-AND-TAKE-YOUR-CHANCES APPROACH:
Sometime the most direct approach is the most effective. The go-for-broke approach can be employed by either the potential strapper or the potential receptive partner. If you intend to sport the strap-on yourself, assemble a dildo and harness rig based on your own preferences and an estimate of what will work well with your partner's body. Put the dildo and harness on under your clothes, arrange a romantic date with your intended, and at an

opportune moment bring her hand to the bulge waiting for her in your jeans.

> I remember looking through a catalog with a learned lover and seeing a woman suck another girl's cock. I exclaimed "I just don't understand... I mean, there aren't any nerve endings in there!" But right then I felt her hard cock against my thigh, and my mouth started watering.

If you fancy yourself on the receiving end, pick out a dildo that suits you, allowing for some extra length for use with a harness. Decide which style of harness you think your partner would prefer. You might want to place the dildo and harness in a box with some condoms and lubricant and wrap them as a gift. Or put the whole kit and caboodle in her dresser drawer and tell her that there is a new outfit awaiting her inside.

If strap-on sex is a new experience for you as a couple, this is a hit-or-miss proposition. If your partner is thrilled by the idea of having strap-on sex with you, then she will be very thrilled indeed. But if she is uncertain about the prospect, such a dramatic entreaty may be too much, and may in fact reverse your progress toward realizing your desires. If you are the prospective strapper and think this might be the case, bring your dildo and harness with you in a bag or coat pocket rather than wearing it. While an erect dildo strapped on and pointing at your girlfriend may intimidate her, a rig folded neatly at the bottom of a toy sack may prove less threatening.

> She came out of the bathroom and I was shocked! She was big, beautiful, and acted like I did this all the time. In reality, I had never done it before, although she would never have known it!

It was the first time I was sexual with her, and she was wearing the dildo and harness. All I could do was laugh. A t that point, the possibility of sex disappeared. I was embarrassed, and she was not pleased.

Improving Communication During Strap-on Sex

TECHNIQUES BORROWED FROM S/M:

Although frequently misunderstood by folks outside their domain, practitioners of sadomasochism (S/M) have much to teach us. A safeword—a word or phrase previously agreed upon to stop the action—can be quite useful when experimenting with strap-on sex. Pick a word other than "no" or "stop," both of which are often uttered in the midst of a hot sexual exchange. Try to choose something that you would never actually say in a sexual context, such as "lizard" or "Watergate." (Though far be it for me to steer your sexuality away from fantasies of either reptiles or Richard Nixon.) Many people use a streetlight system wherein red equals stop, yellow indicates slow down, and green means full speed ahead.

Blindfolds, another S/M staple, can also be of use during strap-on play. Not only can a blindfold increase the level of expectation and heighten sensory awareness for the receptive partner, but they are a godsend for the intrepid novice strapper. If you fear that your preparations will resemble the Marx Brothers more than Marc Anthony, try blindfolding your partner to help alleviate your self-consciousness.

THE MASTERS AND JOHNSON TECHNIQUE:

A technique developed by sexologists at the Masters and Johnson Institute requires that you and your partner set aside an hour or so to conduct a scientific survey. Focus on one partner at a time, with the other taking on the role of sexual scientist. The scientist's job is to caress her partner in a variety of ways, gently at first, and then increasing the level of stimulation if the partner is receptive. The subject's job is to respond to these sensations by assigning each of them a rating based on the amount of pleasure or discomfort he experiences: -3 for highly unpleasant, -2 for somewhat unpleasant, -1 for slightly unpleasant, 0 for neutral, 1 for slightly pleasurable, 2 for somewhat pleasurable, and 3 for highly pleasurable. This exercise can easily be adapted to strap-on sex, both as a means of learning more about the dimensions of your partner's vagina or anus prior to strap-on sex, and during dildo penetration itself. You may feel somewhat awkward during this data-gathering session, but the research will prove beneficial later on.

> I say "Mmmm," when it works and nothing when it doesn't.

> For me, the most important part of sexual communication is when I look into my husband's eyes as we make love—whether it's strap-on sex or another act altogether.

When Trying Something New, Combine It With the Tried and True

This nugget is one of my favorite instructional standbys, and I have found it to be true in many different sexual scenarios. To put this idea into play, simply combine strap-on sex with another sexual activity that you and your partner currently enjoy. Choose an element of your sexual repertoire about which you both feel comfortable and confident. For example, if you and your partner love oral sex, include it in your sex session prior to either revealing the presence of a packed strap-on rig or slipping off to the bathroom and into a rig you have previously stashed underneath the sink. Then—don't use it! Instead, relax into oral sex as usual. After you've enjoyed that venture, introduce the new toy. This process will help loosen your inhibitions and reduce any performance anxiety around strap-on sex by allowing you and your partner to enjoy the sexual gratification and intimacy associated with a familiar pleasure. In addition, you will likely lessen any performance anxiety you may have felt, since much of the focus on your new strap-on skills will have dissipated.

> Bringing it up with a partner who wants to please is not hard. I just tell her that I want her to pump me hard when she is fucking me with her fingers, and then I tell her I want it harder—and I have just the right thing to do the job!

Bibliography
and Resources

14

Bibliography

101 Nights of Great Sex by Laura Corn (Park Avenue Publishing, 1996).

Anal Pleasure and Health: A Guide for Men and Women, by Jack Morin (Down There Press, 1998).

Best Lesbian Erotica 2000, selected and introduced by Joan Nestle, Tristan Taormino, series editor (Cleis Press, 2000).

Doing It for Daddy: Short Sexy Fiction About a Very Forbidden Fantasy, edited by Pat Califia (Alyson Publications, 1994).

Drag King Book: A First Look, by Del LaGrace Volcano and Judith "Jack" Halberstam (Serpents Tail, 1999).

Female Masculinity, by Judith Halberstam (Duke University Press, 1998).

The Femme's Guide to the Universe, by Shar Rednour (Alyson Publications, 2000).

FTM: Female-to-Male Transsexuals in Society, by Holly Devor (Indiana University Press, 1997).

The Good Vibrations Guide to the G-Spot, by Cathy Winks (Down There Press, 1998).

Good Vibrations: The Complete Guide to Vibrators, by Joani Blank (Down There Press, 1989).

The Leather Daddy and the Femme: An Erotic Novel, by Carol Queen (Cleis Press, 1998).

Leatherwomen III: The Clash of the Cultures, edited by Laura Antoniou (Masquerade Books, 1998).

Macho Sluts, by Pat Califia (Alyson Publications, 1989).

Melting Point, by Pat Califia (Alyson Publications, 1996).

The New Good Vibrations Guide to Sex, by Cathy Winks and Anne Semans (Cleis Press, 1997).

The Persistent Desire: A Femme–Butch Reader, edited by Joan Nestle (Alyson Publications, 1992).

PoMoSexuals. Challenging Assumptions about Gender and Identity, edited by Carol Queen and Lawrence Schimel (Cleis Press, 1997).

Repetitive Strain Injury: A Computer User's Guide, Emil Pascarelli and Deborah Quilter (John Wiley and Sons, 1994).

Sex Changes: The Politics of Transgenderism, by Pat Califia (Cleis Press, 1997).

Susie Sexpert's Lesbian Sex World, by Susie Bright (Cleis Press, 1990, 1998).

Transgender Warriors: Making History from Joan of Arc to Dennis Rodman, by Leslie Feinberg (Beacon, 1997).

Trans Liberation: Beyond Pink or Blue, by Leslie Feinberg (Beacon, 1998).

The Ultimate Guide to Anal Sex for Women, by Tristan Taormino (Cleis Press, 1997).

Virgin Territory and *Virgin Territory 2,* edited by Shar Rednour (Masquerade Books, 1996, 1997).

The Whole Lesbian Sex Book: A Passionate Guide for All of Us, by Felice Newman (Cleis Press, 1999).

Magazines

Anything That Moves
Bisexual quarterly.
2261 Market St., Ste. #496,
San Francisco, CA 94114
www.anythingthatmoves.com
info@anythingthatmoves.com

Bad Attitude
P.O. Box 39110, Cambridge, MA 02139

Black Sheets
Pansexual 'zine.
www.queernet.org/BlackBooks

Diva
The U.K.'s lesbian publication.
116–134, Bayham St.,
London, England NW1 0BA
www.gaytimes.co.uk
diva@gaytimes.co.uk

Lesbians On the Loose
Australia's lesbian magazine.
P.O. Box 1099,
Darlinghurst, Australia 1300
www.lotl.com
lotl@lotl.com

Lespress
Germany's lesbian magazine.
Kaiser-Karl-Ring 57, D-53111 Bonn
www.lespress.de
info@lespress.de

On Our Backs
The Best of Lesbian Sex
HAF Enterprises
3415 César Chavez, Ste. 101,
San Francisco, CA 94110
www.gfriends.com/onourbacks
staff@gfriends.con

Skin Two
The world's leading fetish magazine.
Unit 63, Abbey Business Centre,
Ingate Place, London SW8 3NS
www.skintwo.co.uk
online@skintwo.co.uk

Transgender Tapestry Magazine
Quarterly magazine "by, for, and about
all things trans, including cross-
dressing, transsexualism, intersexuality,
FTM, MTF, butch, femme, drag kings
and drag queens, androgyny, female
and male impersonation, and more."
IFGE, P.O. Box 540229.
Waltham, MA 02545
www.ifge.org/tgmag/tgmagtop.htm
editor@ifge.org

Whap! Magazine
(323) 782-WHAP phone
(323) 653-WHAP fax
www.whapmag.com
Campy, retro-style magazine for
heterosexual female dommes and male
submissives

Zaftig!
Sex for the well rounded.
54 Boynton St., 1st Floor,
Boston, MA 02130
www.xensei.com/users/zaftig/home.htm
zaftig@xensei.com

Retail and Mail Order

Adam and Gillian's
Sensual Whips and Toys
The Utopian Network
PO Box 1146, New York, NY 10156
(631) 842-1711

Aslan Leather
A woman-owned manufacturer of
leather, rubber, and vinyl gear,
including dildo harnesses.
Box 102, Stn. B,
Toronto, ON M5T 2T3, Canada
(416) 306.0462
www.AslanLeather.com
aslan@interlog.com

A Woman's Touch
600 Williamson St.,
Madison, WI 53703
(608) 250-1928
www.a-womans-touch.com/
wmstouch@midplains.net

Blowfish
Mail-order catalog of toys, books,
magazines, videos, and safer-sex
supplies.
P.O. Box 411290,
San Francisco CA 94141
Tel. (800) 325-2569
Tel. (415) 252-4340
Fax (415) 252-4349
www.blowfish.com
blowfish@blowfish.com

Come As You Are
701 Queen St. W.,
Toronto, ON, M6J 1E6, Canada
Toll-free: (877) 858-3160
(416) 504-7934
www.comeasyouare.com
mail@comeasyouare.com

Cupid's Treasure
3519 North Halstead,
Chicago, IL 60657
(773) 348-3884

Eros Boutique
581A Tremont St., Boston, MA 02118
http://www.erosboutique.com

Fetishes Boutique
704 S. 5th St., Philadelphia PA 19147
Phone: (215) 829-4986
Toll-free: (877) 2CORSET
www.fetishesboutique.com

Good for Her
175 Harbord St.,
Toronto, ON Canada M5S 1H3
Toll-free: (877) 588-0900
(416) 588-0900
www.goodforher.com
whats@goodforher.com

Good Vibrations

Stores:

1210 Valencia St.,
San Francisco, CA 94110
(415) 974-8980

2504 San Pablo Ave.,
Berkeley, CA 94702
(510) 841-8987

Mail-order:

938 Howard St., Ste. #101, San
Francisco, CA 94103
(800) 289-8423
(415) 974-8990
www.goodvibes.com
goodvibe@well.com

Grand Opening!
318 Harvard St., Ste. #32, Arcade Bldg.,
Coolidge Corner, Brookline, MA 02446
Toll-free ordering line: (877) 731-2626
Tel. (617) 731-2626
FAX (617) 731-2693
www.grandopening.com
grando@grandopening.com

Greedy Dyke Productions
Harness manufacturer.
2400 Rio Grande NW #1-110,
Albuquerque, NM 87104
www.nmia.com/~misskell/gdprod.html
misskell@nmia.com

Intimacies
28 Center Street,
Northampton, MA 01060
(413)582-0709 (V/TTY)
www.intimaciesonline.com/

Jaguar Adult Books
4057 18th St., San Francisco CA 94114
(415) 863-4777

Lovecraft
63 Yorkville Ave.,
Toronto, ON Canada M5R 1B7
(416)923-7331

2200 Dundas Street East
Mississauga, ON Canada L4X 2V3
(905)276-5772
www.lovecraft.inter.net

Mercury Mail Order
4084 18th St., San Francisco CA 94114
(415) 621-1188

Nice-N-Naughty Online Toy Store
www.nice-n-naughty.com

The Pleasure Chest
7733 Santa Monica Blvd.,
West Hollywood, CA 90046
(323) 650-1022
www.thepleasurechest.com

Pleasure Palace
277 Dalhousie St.,
Ottawa ON Canada K1N 7E5
(613) 789-7866

Pleasure Place
1710 Connecticut Ave. NW,
Washington, DC 20009
www.pleasureplace.com

Purple Passion
242 West 16th St.,
New York, NY 10010
(212) 807-0486
www.purplepassion.com

SH!
22 Coronet St., London N1, U.K.
(0171) 613 5458

Stormy Leather
1158 Howard St.,
San Francisco, CA 94103
(415) 626-1672
www.stormyleather.com

Toys in Babeland
(800) 658-9119
www.babeland.com
biglove@babeland.com
Stores:

711 E. Pike St., Seattle, WA 98122
(206) 328-2914

94 Rivington St., New York, NY 10002
(212) 375-1701

Venus Envy
1598 Barrington St., Halifax, Nova
Scotia, Canada B3J 1Z6
(902) 422-0004
www.venusenvy.ns.ca

Vixen Creations
Women-owned and -operated
manufacturer of hand-made silicone
dildos and plugs.
1004 Revere, Ste. B-49,
San Francisco, CA 94124
(415) 822-0403
www.vixencreations.com
VixenSi@sirius.com

Womyn's Ware
896 Commercial Dr.,
Vancouver, BC, V5L 3Y5, Canada
Toll-free (888) WYM-WARE (996-9273)
(604) 254-2543
www.womynsware.com
info@womynsware.com

Xandria Collection
Vibrators, dildos, lingerie, leather,
videos, books, and more.
165 Valley Dr., Brisbane, CA 94005
(800) 242-2823
(415) 468-3812
www.xandria.com
info@xandria.com

Index

15

About the Author

KARLYN LOTNEY is a sex educator and writer. Known to thousands of readers as Fairy Butch, Lotney dispenses sex advice in *Curve* magazine and on PlanetOut.com. She has written for *On Our Backs, Paramour,* Sidewalk.com and other publications. She teaches sexuality workshops to both women and men, and is the resident dildo expert at Good Vibrations, the "clean well-lighted" sex toy store. Lotney is the host of San Francisco's popular cabaret In Bed with Fairy Butch.